Herbs Gone Wild!

Ancient Remedies Turned Loose

Herbs Gone Wild!
Ancient Remedies Turned Loose

Printed in the United States of America
ISBN: 978-0-9839155-4-6

Cover Design by: Diane Kidman

Published by: carp(e) libris press, LLC

Visit the Author Website at:
www.DianeKidman.com

Table of Contents

Introduction

Our grandmothers would want us to know — our ancestral grandmothers, the ones from so long ago that our only proof they existed is our own reflection in the mirror. Those women would want us to know how to depend on the natural world as they once did, finding healing in the plants and trees. They didn't get to run to the pharmacy for a box of cold capsules. They didn't have bottles of anti-inflammatories, pink bottles of bismuth, blue bottles of liquid that stops everything, including you, so you sleep through the flu.

They also didn't have infant pain reliever recalls, they didn't worry about red dye #5 making children's cough syrup look like candy, and they didn't have to lay awake at night wondering whether or not they should have started their three-year-old on an antibiotic prescription for the sniffles.

No doubt they spent many sleepless nights thinking about the other scary things they had to endure. Sure, our ancestors had afflictions to fear that we don't give a second thought to anymore. These days, the flu is rarely deadly. But it's not because we have a bottle of flu medicine in the cupboard. And thank God for doctors who can undo our health catastrophes when the flu does go haywire.

But what we've lost touch with is the ability to care for ourselves, the everyday dings and bangs, sneezes and hacks that for grandmother was second nature. One hundred years ago, she could probably go to a pharmacy if she lived in the city, but she'd purchase packages of dried herbs and bottles of herbal tinctures. That's what pharmacies sold. Herbs.

1

Less than 200 years ago, she knew how to go find the stuff herself. It grew in her garden. It hung in bundles drying near the hearth. It filled jars and burlap bags, it bubbled on the stove whenever a family member was in need of what she almost instinctively knew, because *her* grandmother taught her.

She knew what to pick the instant her son tripped and scraped his knee. A kiss on a boo boo was still the treatment of choice, but a poultice of yarrow or comfrey was sure to follow after.

These are the things we'd do well to remember. Simple, effective, and close to home.

Our grandmothers would want us to know.

How to Use This Book

Herbs Gone Wild! is a collection of remedies that are mostly for common ailments, acute conditions that aren't here for the long haul, and first aid type "everybody experiences them" sort of things. I can tell you what to take for a stress headache. I can't suggest you treat a brain tumor with a chamomile flower.

I am not a doctor but an herbalist, which means I surround myself with herbs at all times; dried, tinctured, fresh. And I use them. I use them on myself, I give them to my family and friends, to people who want them and who benefit from them.

I'm a person who loves herbs, who makes studying them a regular part of life, and who will eat just about any plant that isn't disgusting or poisonous. (Okay, I will eat the ones that are disgusting. But I avoid the poisonous ones. Herbalist rule #1: Don't eat the poisonous ones.)

PLEASE NOTE: Serious ailments require a doctor or proper medical attention. *Herbs Gone Wild!* is filled with suggestions and is not meant to diagnose or treat serious conditions that are best left to the doctors. I also ask that you keep this in mind: If it appears to be a minor problem but you have a nagging feeling that something's not right, go with your gut and get thee to a doctor. Don't wait around on a persistent high fever, serious injury, or visions of angels before you stop treating yourself and find the proper help.

If you just need a little help to get through the common cold, however, or if you have a horrible toothache and can't get to the dentist until Monday morning, then I'm your girl and this is your book.

Most of what follows are remedies that rely on easy-to-find herbs. You don't have to be a master herb gardener, you don't have to hunt down the elusive pipsissewa in the woods. Unless you want to. You can, however, find these herbs easily in commerce, whether it be at your local health food store or from a reputable online source.

If you want to find a remedy quickly, or if you'd like to find out what uses there are for a particular herb, I recommend reading the book straight through while bookmarking the pages you like, especially my witty banter for later perusal and quoting at dinner parties; in essence, highlight the good stuff.

For the more adventurous of you, I've included some how-to's at the end of this book, including how to make your own salve and tincture, and how to properly make an herbal tea for medicinal use. There you'll also find a list of all the herbs mentioned in this book in a section called the Herbal Medicine Chest. It also supplies you with dosages for tincture and tea, which makes it great for quick reference.

IMPORTANT: Included in the Herbal Medicine Chest is a conversion for calculating dosages for children. Please do not give children the full dosages within this book, and always be wary before administering any alternative medications with children. While most of the herbs discussed in *Herbs Gone Wild!* are indeed okay for most kids, there's always someone who's allergic to something, even things we assume no one could possibly be allergic to.

You'll probably find that reading the book straight through before relying on it as a reference tool will help give you a better overall picture of the herbs included here. In many ways, it's pretty tough to discuss herbs one symptom at a time, and you'll notice several herbs come up again and again. That's because one herb does so much and can tackle what

4

may appear at first blush to be a whole myriad of unrelated issues. But that's part of their beauty.

Now it's time to prop up the old photos of your grandmas-gone-by, brew yourself a cup of chamomile tea, and enjoy the ride. You may just find a part of yourself you didn't even know was missing.

Cold, Flu, & Virus

Picture this: I'm sitting in the crowded optometrist waiting room, my son on my lap. Wall-to-wall children all waiting for an eye exam. In walks a couple with their 11-year-old girl. She's in her pajamas and her slippers, and she has a nasty case of bed head. Her cough rivals the sound of a dachshund after a squirrel. Why would a parent bring their sick child into close contact with so many healthy children? Did she really need her eyeglass prescription updated that day? The poor kid looked like she needed to be nowhere but in bed. As soon as my son and I got home, I cracked out my bottle of echinacea extract and slipped it into my son's every beverage. He really digs the stuff. I fed him large portions of broccoli and cranberry relish, both loaded in vitamin C. Fortunately, he likes that too. Two days later, he woke up crying with a slight fever. I immediately started him on some homeopathic cold tablets. He sneezed twice. Cold over. Are you seeing what I'm missing here? Okay, I'll clue you in. I did not take echinacea. I did not eat large quantities of broccoli and cranberry. I did not own homeopathic cold tablets for myself. I caught a cold with a heinous barking cough. I eventually took care of myself, but even though I did right by my son, I should have done it for the whole family. I still screw that up sometimes, but I'm learning – and I hope you will too. Because you never know when you'll have a run-in with a pajama-clad child coughing like a mad dachshund.

Multi-Symptom Remedies

Elderberry Syrup

For a decadent remedy to take at the onset of colds and flu, you can try this elderberry syrup. I'm considering planting elderberry (*Sambucus nigra*) in my yard just so I can harvest the berries to make a new batch each year.

Collect the berries (no exact measuring required here, but about a cup is a good place to start), place them in a pan, and smash them well. Simmer on very low heat and continue to smash so you can release as much juice as possible. Once you've released the juice, strain out the crushed berry material and measure the juice. Add an equal amount of honey to the juice, along with a pinch of cinnamon, clove, or ginger (according to your tastes). Add a few drops of lemon and 20% alcohol. For instance, if you have 10 ounces of juice, you'd want to add 2 ounces of alcohol. Something like vodka would work just fine. You can take this syrup liberally as soon as you feel the symptoms of cold or flu sneaking up. Take it often. This is one time you won't mind taking your medicine.

If you enjoy the heat of a spicy pepper, you'll be happy to hear it's good for you. Cayenne (*Capsicum spp.*) taken at the beginning of a cold will help you build up resistance, making it easier to fight the virus. Add fresh cayenne to your dinner or sprinkle dried cayenne on just about anything, or if you're really brave, just eat the darned thing whole. Don't overdo it, of course. You don't want a burning stomach in place of the cold symptoms.

A Tea for the Cold

Blend two parts dried stinging nettle (*Urtica dioica*) to one part dried licorice root (*Glycyrrhiza glabra*) and one part dried rose hips (*Rosaceae*). The nettle is loaded with vitamins and minerals, licorice root sweetens the tea and aids with sore throats and coughs, and rose hips are a good source of vitamin C. Drink as needed.

Another tea you can rely on to help you through a cold would be yarrow (*Achillea millefolium*). It's useful in offering relief for cold and flu symptoms, fevers, and respiratory infections. Yarrow grows abundantly just about anywhere, so it's easy to gather in fields or grow in your own garden. Use the dried flowering tops and dried leaves off the top ⅓ of the plant. You can prepare a standard tea and drink 2 to 4 ounces at a time up to 5 times daily. If you prefer, you can take it as a tincture, 10 to 40 drops, up to 5 times a day.

The Sore Throat

Your little one has a scratchy throat and doesn't want those sticky five-year-old cough drops that sit in the bottom of your purse. Instead, squeeze ½ a lemon in a glass of mineral water (or tap if that's what you've got handy), add a large spoon of honey, and stir until it dissolves as best as you can.

Alternatively, you can prepare a strong ginger tea, adding some honey and lemon juice. When it's cool add a little mineral water for a soothing fizz. Both of these remedies do a good job of breaking up lung goop, too. The ginger is warming and soothing to irritated lungs and can bring down a fever by sweating it out. It also reduces headache, nausea, and vomiting. Either as a warm tea or a fizzy ginger ale, it's an overall nice choice for natural cold and flu treatment.

Ginger tea bags are readily available, or you may choose to go with fresh ginger root, something fairly common at most grocery stores. To prepare it fresh, peel a large chunk of root (maybe 6 inches or so), chop it roughly, and toss it in a saucepan. Fill the pan with water (5 or 6 cups) and simmer the water down about halfway. At this point you can strain out the ginger and add honey to taste. This tea is very spicy! A spicy ginger tea is indeed delicious, but it's also fantastic if you allow it to cool and water it down with a bit of mineral or soda water.

Licorice tea is also good for sore throats and for certain coughs, especially the irritating, scratchy ones that make public speaking seem like a horrifying idea. Licorice root (*Glycyrrhiza glabra*) is good for lung ailments such as bronchitis. Kids like licorice tea as well because it's mild and naturally sweet, nothing like Grandpa's overpowering licorice candies.

To enjoy the tea, use about a teaspoon of dried licorice root in a cup of almost boiling water. Let it steep for about 10 to 20 minutes, depending on how potent a flavor you prefer. (Kids usually like it on the weaker side.) A note of caution, however: Licorice root is safe overall, but it's not for pregnant women or people with high blood pressure. Use it when you need it, don't when you don't.

To make your own sore throat spray, try taking 1 ounce of distilled water, 1 ounce glycerin, and 15 to 30 drops of yerba mansa (*Anemopsis*) tincture. Place it in a spray bottle and shake well before use. It's best to refrigerate this mixture so it will last a few days; hopefully by then, your sore throat will be history. The spray stimulates mucous secretions and is antimicrobial. It can also double as a spray for sore, swollen gums.

Tonsillitis

A gargle made from a cup of tepid purified water and about 20 drops of goldenseal tincture can be used as needed for the relief of tonsillitis. I am the first to admit that goldenseal (*Hydrastis canadensis*) will not be a favorite with the kiddies. It tastes pretty awful, in my opinion. But my husband uses it without cringing, so it's possible. And, hey, it works.

Coughing

A single teaspoon of honey is just as effective as the average over-the-counter cough syrup, as proven by recent studies. And it doesn't contain synthetic alcohols, artificial colors and flavors, or nasty things that make kids buy and sell it on street corners. The best part? You get to take it as often as you feel like it.

You can also try your hand at making some homemade cough syrups. They're fun to make, and some of them don't taste awful. Some do. I'll leave it up to you to decide which is which.

Homemade Natural Cherry Cough Syrup

2 cups cherries (organic is best)
2 cups honey
a lemon
water

Put the cherries in a pan and just cover them with water. Add the honey and some lemon slices – at least half the lemon. Simmer carefully until the cherries are completely soft and you're able to remove the pits. Also remove the lemon. Place the mixture into a jar and store it in the refrigerator. You can use several tablespoons whenever you need it.

A little hint here: Since cherries are available in summertime and colds and coughing are available through fall and winter, you can actually freeze this and other liquefied herbal remedies in ice cubes to thaw out for later use. I do it all the time. It's fun to send guests to the freezer for ice, then watch them jump when they notice the cubes are varying shades of green and brown.

Diane's Homemade Cough Syrup

1 cup purified water
1 tsp. dried ground ginger or ½-inch peeled, finely chopped ginger
½ tsp. dried licorice root (*Glycyrrhiza glabra*)
½ tsp. dried horehound (*Marrubium*)
½ cup honey
A dash or two cayenne pepper

Take water in a saucepan and add dried ground ginger or fresh ginger. Heat water to a low simmer. Simmer until the water is reduced to half, then turn off the heat. Add dried licorice root and dried horehound to a tea ball and steep in the ginger tea, covered, for 20 to 30 minutes. (If you like, leave the ginger root in the pan for strong ginger flavor. It's more soothing to a sore throat and cough when the ginger is on the stronger side.) Remove the tea ball and strain out the ginger. If the tea has cooled, return it to the pan and heat it up just a little. Turn the heat off and add honey and stir until totally dissolved. Add cayenne, as much as you can stand. Wait for the mixture to cool and store in an amber bottle or jar with a tight-fitting lid. Keep refrigerated or freeze. Good for a week in the fridge. This works great for congested lungs.

Fever

Too often we freak out when a fever occurs. But don't forget, a fever means the body is working hard to fight the virus. High fevers and lasting fevers always warrant a call to the doc, especially with kids. And always call whenever your parenting radar says, "Hey, this just doesn't feel right."

Only break a fever with herbs if the fever is 103° or lower for adults, 101.5° and lower for kids. If the fever is higher than that, you don't want heating herbs that will temporarily spike the fever even higher before it calms it. To break a fever, you can try peppermint or ginger tea, or eat dinner with lots of extra garlic. For the brave at heart, nibbling on a raw clove of garlic will conk out that fever faster than you can say, "Why do I have the sweats?" It will also chase away vampires and most family members.

For a fever without the sweats, you can drink a yarrow (*Achillea millefolium*) tea which will dilate your peripheral blood vessels and bring down the fever, eliminating some of your symptoms as it goes. Take 2 to 4 ounces up to 5 times a day.

Boneset (*Eupatorium perfoliatum*) tincture or tea is the perfect choice for hot, sweaty fevers due to a viral infection. Pair that fever with aches and pains, inflammation, splitting headaches, and other similar classic flu symptoms, and you're ripe for boneset. Although it's specifically good for hot, sweaty flues, it'll help for the dry fever as well. Put 20 to 40 drops of the fresh plant tincture in hot water and take up to 4 times a day; alternatively, you can prepare a boneset tea and drink 2 to 6 ounces up to 3 times a day.

Stuffy Nose

When it comes to remedies for the stuffy nose, I've got more up my sleeve than just a wad of tissue. Most of these remedies are safe for any age.

Boil 4 cups of water with ¼ cup lemon thyme and inhale the steam. For little ones, use very close supervision and inhale with them. Then you'll be certain the steam isn't too hot or too powerful. Or try ½ cup of apple cider vinegar and ½ cup of water. Boil and inhale the steam, same as with the lemon thyme concoction.

This is one of my favorite stuffy nose remedies – the neti pot. This is a solution for older children and adults, and although the neti pot may seem like an unpleasant idea, it's actually the most effective way of relieving a stuffy nose that I know. The neti pot looks like a squat watering can made of ceramic. Using warm distilled water (not too hot!) and about ½ teaspoon of Kosher salt and ¼ teaspoon baking soda, you flush out your sinuses by leaning over the sink, tipping your head slightly, and pouring into one nostril. The water magically comes out the other nostril, thus giving your sinuses a full cleansing. Trust me – it doesn't hurt at all. If it did, I'd never use one. You can purchase neti pots online, in health food stores, and even in some pharmacies. They come with more detailed instructions, so follow those carefully and you'll enjoy breathing easily once again.

A few drops of eucalyptus oil in a humidifier that has a special reservoir for oils can clear not only stuffy noses but a congested chest. Or mix a few drops of the oil in about ½ oz. of olive or sweet almond oil for a chest rub. For very small children and babies, be sure the room is properly ventilated, and go easy on the eucalyptus. It can be done, but babies and young children are much more sensitive to scent and need very little oil for it to be effective. Lavender or rosemary oil are other nice choices.

Another little-known favorite of mine takes some forethought in the early summer. We've all seen ox-eye daisy (*Chrysanthemum leucanthemum*) in fields and on roadsides; maybe you even grow it in your garden. As long as you can properly identify it, and as long as you can pick some from a safe, pesticide-free area (without secreting it from your neighbor's garden, even if she does grow a ton), snag handfuls of blooms and dry them well before storing them in a clean, dry jar with a tight-fitting lid. When a stuffy nose comes along, make a mug of tea with a heaping teaspoon of dried blooms. In about 30 minutes or less, a stuffed nose will be clear, and it should stay that way effectively for 4 to 6 hours, same as any cold capsule – without the side effects. This works best with swollen nasal passages or a drippy nose. Drink a cup of the tea up to 4 times a day.

This next remedy I learned from herbalist Ed Smith of HerbPharm. I interviewed him for a podcast on my blog dkMommy Spot a couple of years back, and he told me this story that I'll not soon forget. You can hear the story in its entirety in that podcast at http://dkmommyspot.com/a-podcast-interview-with-herbal-ed/. To give you the story in a nutshell, a woman had an infant who was congested, so much so that she couldn't breastfeed the baby. Not knowing what to do, the concerned parents took their child to Dr. John Christopher who ground some fresh horseradish (*Armoracia*), placed a wad of it in the palm of his hand, and cupped his hand over the baby's nose and mouth. After a few inhalations of the fumes from the potent root and a bit of coughing, the baby sneezed out what was a very large and cleansing sneeze, ultimately releasing all the goop clogging his sinuses. After a couple more monster sneezes, the baby's breathing was restored to normality and lunch was back on.

15

I love that story because it proves once again how powerful herbs can be and how they're a true natural alternative to the medications with side effects. Just think. Those parents couldn't have used anything over the counter with such a young child. They also needed that baby breathing normally right away. Having some herbal knowledge like this at your disposal is invaluable.

Infection

Whether the bronchitis is getting the better of you or the cold has progressed into a nasty sinus infection, your first instinct may be to rush for the antibiotics. I'm not going to tell you to forgo antibiotics when necessary. Yes, it's true that there still are doctors out there who will crack out the prescription pad over a mere sniffle or a virus, against which antibiotics are useless. But infections must be dealt with, and there are some natural alternatives that you may want to consider.

When my son was about six months old, he got his first cold. It lasted a whopping 2 days. Mine lasted a week, complete with rising temperature, coughing, splitting headaches, and a sinus infection. I finally dragged myself to the doctor. He said, "Dear, you've got an infection in your lungs, your sinuses, and both ears. Time for that antibiotic." I told him I was breastfeeding and didn't want my baby to have to take the prescription through me. I said I'd prefer to go with a strong round of acidophilus from my health food store. Being one of those rare docs that appreciates natural remedies and actually knows what I'm talking about when I mention dandelion greens like it's medicine, he said, "Alright, but you have to promise me that if it doesn't start to clear up in a couple of days, that you'll get this prescription filled, breastfeeding or no."

I got the strongest acidophilus I could find from my local health food store, and within 2 days, the fever was gone.

Within about the same timeframe an antibiotic would have cleared me up, the acidophilus did the same thing, and without taking my immune system down with it.

Acidophilus has proven itself to me over and over again, eradicating some of the nastiest of sinus infections, ear infections, and bronchial infections I've ever had. Am I telling you to never take an antibiotic again? Heavens, no. But know your natural options because they do exist.

My best advice when choosing a good acidophilus is to go with what is in the refrigerated section. Always check for the expiration date. These are live cultures (or at least they should be), and if it's expired, you're not getting your money's worth. Try out a brand or two when infection isn't so bad, or when you have a mild problem, say, the very beginning of a sinus infection. If the infection continues to worsen, you may not have a brand that works for you.

I've heard herbalist Michael Moore state that everyone's a little different when it comes to which brands work for them. He recommended starting out with the cheaper brands first, moving your way up until you find the most effective one. Unfortunately for me, the most effective one is also the most expensive. But it's all worth it in the end. I have avoided numerous trips to the doctor and countless prescriptions, not to mention all the side effects that come along with repeated bouts of antibiotics.

Immunostimulants

Whether you're building up your kids' constitutions to avoid catching viruses at school, or you're sick and tired of getting sick and tired from your coworkers' colds, having a good immunostimulant or two as part of your herbal medicine chest is a fantastic idea. These herbs will help you to beef up your defenses so it's tougher for those viruses to set up camp.

17

I can't go without mentioning echinacea *(Echinacea angustifolia* or *purpurea)* right from the get-go. Echinacea can be taken before your kids even head back to school — say about a week or two before, 5 or 10 drops a day in some water for prevention —and can be continued right through the school year, if you so choose. I've heard talk about taking a break from echinacea so your body won't "get used to" the herb. Not necessary. I've also heard grumblings that taking echinacea doesn't allow your body to build up its own defenses. Simply not true. It's quite the opposite, in fact. Echinacea helps your body build up its own defenses, which is what makes this herb such a powerhouse.

If you didn't remember to start up that echinacea before cold and flu season has begun, you can still grab some as soon as you feel those first signs of illness. Other potential herbs at this point would be: balsa wood *(Ochroma pyramidale)*, arbor vitae *(Thuja spp.)*, marshmallow *(Althaea officinalis)*, or even arnica *(Arnica spp.)* These are all great immunostimulants. Even if life is getting particularly stressful and you've been wearing yourself thin, making you the perfect target for a virus, it's good to have these herbal friends at hand. Take them when you're burning the candle at both ends so you don't find yourself stuck in bed later.

If you're the sort who gets several colds a year, or even if you're prone to herpes outbreaks, you might want to give balsamroot *(Balsamorhiza)* a try. It's similar in effect to echinacea, with the added benefit of being a bit heating, so it knocks the chilly out of you while making your immune system stronger. It's a wee bit bitter as tea, so if that bothers you, try the tincture of the fresh or dry root, 20 to 50 drops in hot water up to 4 times a day.

Chicken Pox & Measles

I remember discovering a large chicken pock on my neck when I was 12 years old. It was Halloween, I was at school putting on my drunken sailor costume for the afternoon party, and I had absolutely no intentions of telling my mother what I'd found. After school, I confided in my little sister and made her pinky swear not to tell. Of course she did. But by then it no longer mattered. I was covered in spots, running a high fever, and in no mood for impersonating an inebriated sailor, even if the charcoaled black eye was a nice touch. (Thanks, Mom.) My sister felt bad for tattling and ended up taking two Halloween buckets out trick-or-treating that evening; one for her, and one for her big sissy. She had so many goodies from well-wishers at the end of the night that she needed help carrying home the booty.

Boneset is perfect for the chicken pox due to its ability to deal with viral infections, and its talent at handling the sort of skin eruptions experienced with chicken pox and measles. Boneset will help bring on the eruptions more quickly, shortening the illness and aiding in curbing any skin damage.

Another herb you can use is pipsissewa (*Chimaphila*), a beautiful little plant that also has the ability to bring the spots on faster, making the duration shorter and more endurable. This plant is good for measles, too. It requires a tea made of 1 tablespoon dried leaves in 1 ½ cup water; simmer for 15 to 20 minutes, and drink the tea 3 times a day. Alternatively, you can use pipsissewa tincture, 20 to 50 drops in water, drunk 4 times a day.

Conjunctivitis & Hordeolum (or Pink Eye and Styes)

Your son wakes up looking like he's coming off a bender, but he's only five. Those bloodshot eyes need some attention, and quick, before he spreads the pink eye to other members of the family. A little goldenseal tea may be just the ticket to restoring his eyes to bright and shining normality. Prepare a wash by making a tea of dried goldenseal (*Hydrastis canadensis*) and waiting for it to completely cool. Use an eyedropper for application. If the child is resistant to the whole eyedropper thing, try a clean cloth dipped in the tea and applied to the eyes. You can repeat this process throughout the day; just be sure to prepare a fresh tea and use a clean cloth each time, to avoid spreading the virus.

Eyebright (*Euphrasia officinalis*) — what a clever name for an herb whose specialty is eye health. It increases circulation to the eye area, therefore making it a wise choice for eradicating conjunctivitis and the like. Make a tea of eyebright (1 tsp. of the herb in 1 cup hot water, steeped for 15 minutes) and use compresses dipped in the tea to hold on the infected eye. Or use the cooled tea for a soothing eyewash.

Echinacea (*Echinacea angustifolium* or *purpurea*) visits us once again. It's safe for kids and babies, and you can use it as a tea, a tincture, or a compress. For compresses, make as a tea (about 1 tsp. steeped in hot water). Or give 30 to 40 drops of the tincture daily, taken internally, to help boost the body's infection-fighting power.

If you're caught off guard and don't have the herbs available when you need them, you can make an eyewash with 1 ½ tsp. baking soda stirred into ¾ cup warm water.

Naturally, if the eye infection doesn't clear up quickly, you'll need to see your pediatrician. But in the meantime, it's nice to have these at-home remedies around for weekends and after-office hours.

Cold Sores

If you're prone to cold sores, you fully understand the horror of waking up with one. Perhaps today is the big job interview. Or maybe you're not in the mood to go to parent-teacher conferences sporting a third eyeball on your upper lip. If you've ever experienced such a thing, you'll want to keep a bottle of gold thread (*Coptis trifolia*) tincture on hand at all times. As soon as you get that first tingle, apply a few drops topically. You can choose to use a strong tea made of the herb instead, although the tincture is more handy. Either way, apply liberally several times a day.

A couple other options are balsamroot (*Balsamorhiza*) or echinacea (*Echinacea angustifolia* or *purpurea*), both of which are perfect for adults who get several outbreaks a year. For the echinacea tincture, use 50 to 60 drops, 3 times a day, taken internally; or drink as a tea, 2 to 4 ounces up to 4 times daily. Balsamroot tincture can be taken 20 to 50 drops up to 4 times a day.

Believe it or not, that old favorite lemon balm (*Melissa officinalis*) is also quite adept in helping with outbreaks. It's both antioxidant and anti-inflammatory, and you can apply the tincture topically. Or take it as a tea as needed to enjoy the smooth, calm sensations of an herbal friend, without grogginess or a hangover. Which may actually help with that interview or with confronting your daughter's math teacher — all without the embarrassing cold sore.

Boils

Anyone who has ever experienced the pain of a boil will be glad to hear there are several herbs that do neat work of relieving this uncomfortable affliction. And since they're common herbs with a multitude of uses, it's easy to see the value of adding them to your herbal medicine chest.

As with cold sores, echinacea (*Echinacea angustifolia* or *purpurea*) tincture can be applied topically, just a few drops to the affected area, several times a day. Echinacea's ability to increase white blood cell count and fight infection makes it a superhero in situations such as this.

Plantain (*Plantago major*) leaves, those weedy things you probably have all over your back yard anyway, can be crushed up and placed on the area as a poultice. (But don't use anything out of your yard if you apply pesticides or fertilizers. Clean plants that grow away from the house only, please.) When I use a plantain poultice for anything, I simply secure the mashed leaves in place with gauze or bandages and change it as needed, at least once a day.

Black walnut (*Juglans major*) tincture is helpful not only for boils, but for tooth abscesses as well. Just apply a few drops of the tincture directly to the affected area several times a day.

Eczema & Psoriasis

Echinacea (*Echinacea angustifolia* or *purpurea*) to the rescue once again. I can't tell you how valuable that herb is as part of the herbal medicine chest for any natural home. In this case, we're talking eczema and psoriasis, skin conditions that ultimately stem from the inside out. Echinacea can help when taken regularly as a tincture (30 to 40 drops up to 5 times a day).

Horse nettle, or bull nettle (*Solanum carolinense*), puts a stop to eczema in a flash. Ten to 40 drops of the tincture taken only one or two times can stop the cycle and clear the skin, and as one sufferer told me, even if it's debilitating eczema. This plant warms from the inside out and will help if your psoriasis or eczema comes along with uncomfortable joint pain.

Another herb to consider for any chronic skin condition, including eczema and psoriasis, is burdock root (*Arctium lappa*). This helpful plant eliminates the toxins from your system that are responsible for your skin issues, and also aids in systemic balance. Take 30 to 90 drops of tincture up to 3 times a day.

First Aid

Perhaps you've already got the little first aid kit with the red cross on the front, and so far it's served you well just sitting there unused and making you feel responsible. I don't recommend giving it the old heave-ho, even if you never crack the thing open. Just keep the contents fresh and updated, and add a few of your own. You'll be surprised how far a few herbs can get you.

Sunburns

No first aid kit needed here. Jumping into cold water is the quickest way to halt the process of a sunburn. Just because you're out of the sun doesn't mean the burning has stopped, so hop into a cold shower or get your child into a cool tub to stop the cooking and start the healing.

To apply something directly to the burn, you've got several choices: Make a spray out of equal parts white vinegar and water. Or make a paste from 1 part baking soda, 1 part cornstarch, and enough water to make a paste to smooth on the burns. Or for a moisturizing, healing remedy, use wheat germ oil to ease the burn and soften the skin. You can also rub cold cucumber slices on the skin, a real comfort for painful sunburns.

Aloe vera gel is one of the best and most common natural solutions for sunburns — or any minor burn, for that matter — but make sure it's completely natural. I can't tell you how many bottles of "natural" aloe I've looked at, only to find an ingredient list a mile long. Aloe vera gel should be just aloe and doesn't need any fancy additives. Look for 100%, and be sure to check the label. If you have an aloe plant at home, and if you only need enough for a burnt face or chest, you can break off a leaf, give it a squeeze, and apply the gel. I often keep the remainder of the leaf in the refrigerator for later use. It keeps for quite awhile, at least until I've burned myself cooking, which is an unfortunate and frequent occurrence.

If you are able to find a good 100% aloe gel, you can boost the healing properties by placing a big glop in a bowl and adding a few drops of lavender oil (*Lavandula angustifolia*). A soothing cool with a comforting scent, most welcome after a long day in the sun.

Remember that the sun is strongest between 10 a.m. and 2 p.m., so try to avoid prolonged exposure during those times. By all means, enjoy the summer heat, have fun with the kids, and don't forget to protect everyone from the sun. But if you do get caught up in all the activity and discover you've gotten too much of a good thing, you know what to do.

Burns

Aloe vera isn't just for sunburns. As I mentioned, I've used it an embarrassing number of times for cooking burns. I hardly think a dinner goes by when I don't absent-mindedly bump something I shouldn't. Could be why I always have aloe plants around. Use the plant for your average burn same as you would the sunburn: Break off a chunk of leaf, squeeze the gel out of the leaf, and apply it to the burn. (I'd suggest running the burn under cold water first, which will stop the skin from continuing to burn.)

If the burn is bad, you should seek the care of a doctor immediately, using some aloe until help can be sought. But for minor burns and blistering, nothing works for healing the pain and redness better than treating it with aloe vera.

Bee & Insect Stings

I'll never forget my first bee sting. I was about four years old, and I received the first natural remedy I can remember. (Except for prune juice, but that's not a fun story.) My mother applied the remedy and some kisses, and all the pain went away.

Shortly afterwards, I was playing in the yard with my mom when she stepped on a yellowjacket and got stung in the arch of her foot. Oh, did it hurt! She started to cry. While she was sitting outside trying to pull out the stubborn bee lodged in her foot, I ran into the kitchen, remembering her remedy. I climbed up on the counter with the help of an old aluminum kitchen chair and got the baking soda, which I mixed with a little water to form a paste. I took it to her, applied it to her foot, and tried to heal her with kisses and hugs. The bee sting went away, but for some reason she cried even harder.

Maybe that's part of the reason I love natural remedies. There's something more personal to them, and I find over and over again that everyone has their own little story, remembering Mom or Grandma preparing something special and mixing it with love to heal the pain.

Poison Ivy

If you've been frolicking in the woods and accidentally find yourself in the poison ivy patch, all is not lost. One of the plants that treats the itch is probably growing nearby.

First off, not too many herbs work well for easing poison ivy. But there's one plant that is heads above the others: jewelweed (*Impatiens capensis*). This isn't something one should purchase in its dried form, as it's better fresh; and it's hard to identify without the telltale orange fairy hat-like flowers in bloom, so it may be tricky to come by, unless you purchase a jewelweed salve or soap product. Nice thing about Jewelweed, you can grow it in your own garden and it's gorgeous. Give it plenty of room, however. It grows tall and full, and I've seen large stands of it in the wild that cover whole banks of lakes and ponds, or lining the edges of woodlands. But it'll be worth the space – the flowers are so lovely, and the seedpods are great fun for kids. That's because the pods explode at the merest touch, ejecting their seeds in a flurry and making everyone jump and laugh. This gives the plant its other common name, Touch-Me-Not.

If you're lucky enough to get a hold of the plant in flower, you can either juice it and apply it topically or gather it up and make a nice salve for later use. I like to take the top 3 inches or so, flower and all, when making the salve. You can read all about how to prepare salves at the end of this book, remember, so if you feel like trying your hand at making your own preparations, you'll end up with a fine remedy that's also good for other rashes and skin irritations.

If making your own salve sounds like too much messing around, another respectable remedy is to prepare the following herbal tea: Mix together about 2 Tbs. wild geranium (*Geranium maculatum*), powdered valerian root (*Valeriana officinalis*), and cinquefoil (*Potentilla*), all in dried form, and place them in about 4 cups of water. Bring to a gentle boil, simmering until the liquid reduces by half. Strain out the herbs, allow the liquid to cool, and use as a compress to soothe the itch of poison ivy. You can store the remainder in the fridge for a few days, or make ice cubes to keep around the rest of the summer.

Cuts & Wounds

Let me paint a little scenario for you. Imagine an herbalist, probably one who looks a lot like me and may even have the same initials, but I'm not sure. She's got a new gardening tool that she's all jacked up to try while wildcrafting in the middle of a field. It's one of those slick all-in-one jobs; part saw, part bowie knife, part little shoveling tool. The Japanese call it a hori hori, which is much more fun to say than "all-in-one gardening tool," so that's what we'll call it. Said herbalist is hacking away at a huge field of yarrow when she slices her thumb clean open. We're talking the kind of cut that hovers for awhile, open and empty before beginning to gush. The oh-so-wise herbalist drops her hori hori to the ground and stares at the cut, mouth agape, wondering what she's gonna do when it begins to gush and she's got nothing more than her other thumb to hold the wound together. Then her learning kicks in, all those hours of book reading and studying. The forehead slapping moment arrives as she looks down at the very large field of yarrow in which she's standing, a bag of fresh cut herb still at her feet, albeit speckled with her own blood.

Yarrow (*Achillea millefolium*). If there's one thing anyone who's spent time around herbs knows, it's that the best thing to seal a cut is fresh yarrow leaves. So our brave herbalist grabs a big leaf, chews it up (insert image of contorted face here), and spits the wad onto the cut, pushing it in for all she's worth. Within about 10 minutes, the wound was completely sealed and the skin had even closed over a bit of leaf, making for a colorful spot to show off to others.

Yarrow is best fresh, and it doesn't need to be in flower to work like this. It's definitely plentiful as a common roadside and field weed, so it's worth it to plant some in your garden. The stuff really takes off and can gobble up a garden if you let it, so pick the location carefully, and hack it back freely for your other herb projects. You can always make a salve with yarrow for year-round use. I keep a tin of yarrow salve in my first aid gear, and it goes wherever that darned hori hori goes. Because I've learned my lesson. From that other herbalist who looks like me.

29

Also, be sure to clean the wound out as best you can before using yarrow because it can trap dirt within the wound.

If you don't have yarrow or other healing herbs available, you might consider this old time remedy instead. During the Civil War, powdered sugar was a common treatment for wounds because of its ability to speed up the healing process. Place powdered sugar on the wound and cover with a bandage. Change the bandage and the powdered sugar regularly to speed healing.

Another quick healer for the open wound is goldenseal (*Hydrastis canadensis*). You can use either tincture or salve. Although tincture may have a bit of a sting to it, the alcohol aids in the killing of germs. Again, you've got to be sure you have a clean wound before application, as the wound will close rapidly.

Comfrey salve is a longtime favorite herbal remedy for skin injuries. Comfrey (*Symphytum officinale*) is easy to come by, whether growing as a prolific weed in the garden or dried in commerce, and a simple salve will prove most useful. If you have it in the garden, grab a few leaves, bruise them, and place them on the injury as a poultice. A tea made from the dried herb and applied with a cloth to the area can also be used.

Sprains

I usually test out my remedies first to see how they work before recommending them. This time, I'll pass. I may be a slave to research, but I draw the line at spraining my own ankle for accuracy in writing. All the same, here are a few ways to treat sprains naturally, or so I am told by fellow ankle-twisting herbalists.

Mix together the white of one egg and enough salt to form a paste. Apply it directly to the sprained area. This is probably the easiest remedy since you won't have to limp far to get eggs and salt. But if you have fresh comfrey leaves, you can apply a poultice. It's also a good time for the comfrey salve, or use a cloth dipped in a tea made from dried comfrey. If you have access to fresh horseradish root, you can grate about 2 Tbs. and mix it with 1 cup of vegetable oil. Simmer it for 10 minutes and strain. This one will last awhile for reapplication. Fresh horseradish is also great for sore joints. And sandwiches.

If you live in the southwest U.S., you probably have lots of sage (*Salvia*) growing wild in your region. But no matter where you live, this is an easy garden plant that requires little attention. Grab a couple handfuls of leaves, squeeze them until bruised, then boil them in a cup of vinegar for five minutes. Soak a cloth in the hot (but not too hot) mixture, squeeze out the excess, and apply the compress to the strain.

St. John's wort oil is a favorite of mine due to its many uses. Its ability to relieve pain, reduce swelling and inflammation, even tend to new bruising and skin irritations makes this a must-have for any natural medicine cabinet. Some herbal oils don't keep very well, but I've had good luck with this one. A glass jar filled with fresh St. John's wort flowers (*Hypericum perforatum*) and covered with sweet almond oil gives you a beautiful red-orange oil in just a couple of weeks. Strain out the flowers and store in a cool, dark location. Mine usually lasts a couple of years in this manner before it's time to make a fresh batch.

Splinters

Prickers, wood slivers, pokey things of all sorts — keep your eyes peeled for plantain, because this mega drawing-out herb can de-splinter without the help of tweezers. Its power is in its ability to pull foreign matter to the surface; it's also helpful in pulling infection out of wounds, bringing boils to a head, even the removal of insect and snake venom. Plantain leaves are just about anywhere humans are, and they're easy to locate at the edge of trails, in your lawn, sprouting out of gravel driveways, etc. Of course, don't ever gather them anywhere there's been weed killers or pesticides applied, or where the environment seems polluted; roadside herbalism is never a good idea. (Think oil, gas, and road salt.) If you have it in your yard (you probably do) and if you don't use chemical treatments on your lawn, you can find this handy plant even in the dead of winter buried under the snow, waiting to serve your splinter needs. Make a poultice of plantain (Plantago *major*) by smashing fresh leaves, or even by chewing some up when you're in a pinch. I personally don't care for the taste of plantain and its ability to eradicate all moisture from the mouth, but I do know some herbalists and wild plant people who enjoy it on sandwiches and salads. If you have a mortar and pestle, you can get the plant material ground well enough to release the juices, which will improve the outcome.

Once the herb is smashed, place a nice glob on the splinter, bug bite, etc., and leave it there. I cover the plantain with a bandage or wrap so it stays in place and doesn't dry out too quickly. For splinters, especially large and/or deep-seated ones, you may need to change the poultice a few times, even over a period of days, before whatever is stuck in you works its way to the surface enough that you can grab it. But even that may not be necessary. Recently, my son got a doozy of a splinter lodged deep into his hand. After trying to remove it ourselves, which involved many tears and no success, I used the "plantain under a bandage" trick that evening. By morning, instead of a deep splinter, there was a bit of a watery blister with the big old hunk of wood sitting in the middle of it, which I was able to wipe away. It really was amazing to see the plantain work so effectively, and my son was relieved indeed. No tweezers!

When doing an herb walk several years ago, one of the participants said she'd used plantain on a good friend who had a piece of shrapnel lodged in his neck. Apparently, the shrapnel was too close to the spine for operating, so the doctors decided to leave it there. She made plantain poultices for her friend and changed them daily until over time they saw the shrapnel work its way to the surface. Is the story true? I can't say. She seemed on the up-and-up, and she did have an awfully nice dog, which always lends credibility, doesn't it? In the end, what grabbed me about that story is the fact that the herbalist leading the walk was surprised – but not surprised. He'd dealt with plantain a lot more than I had at that point, and he seemed to see it as a reasonable expectation of the plant's power.

Mosquito Bites

Again, plantain (*Plantago major*) is our friend here. Easy to find around any mosquito-infested campsite, and you won't have to chew it this time. Just snag a leaf and rub it on the skin until it turns your skin green. My favorite mosquito bite eradicator!

Jellyfish Stings

I know what you're thinking. I saw that episode of Friends too, and I'm simply not going there. Since the summer months mean lots of vacations and beach time, you should know a few options to treat a jellyfish sting, and one that's not offered by Joey and Chandler. (And in case you missed that one, the remedy involved urinating on the sting. Ick.)

If you're going to be swimming in an area known to have jellyfish, take a small bottle of vinegar to the beach. Pouring it slow and steady onto the sting for a good 30 seconds can neutralize the pain from many varieties of jellyfish. Afterwards, you can carefully pull off those nasty little tentacles. But don't remove them until after you've neutralized the tentacles with the vinegar — at least not with your bare hands. You might just get yourself stung again. You can scrape them with the edge of a shell or a credit card instead, if you're wary.

You can also use a mixture of water and baking soda, 50/50, to pour on the sting in the same manner as with the vinegar solution. If you're fresh out of vinegar and there's no baking soda sitting around the beach, salt water from the ocean will do. Immersing the sting in hot water can help, as can cold water, but hot seems to be more effective.

If you or someone you're with has been stung by a jellyfish, you need to seek medical attention right away if the following signs of a rare allergic reaction are present: difficulty breathing, nausea, swelling around the mouth and/or the stung limb, wheezing, chest pain, stomach cramps, or dizziness.

Call the National Marine and Freshwater Envenomation Hotline if you are in any doubt: 1-888/232-8635. A great phone number for the beach bag — right next to the vinegar bottle.

So there, Joey and Chandler, don't you feel foolish? Coulda been a lot easier. (By the way, their solution may actually make the sting worse, so no need to try it.)

Anti-Bacterial Alternatives

The question continues to resurge: "Is antibacterial soap unsafe?" Perhaps you recall it was a pretty big news flash several years ago in regards to how the use of antibacterial soaps could make our bodies more resistant to antibiotics. More recently, they've been talking about the actual ingredients, namely triclosan. An article from Reuters in 2009 stated, "The FDA noted that there was no evidence that triclosan could be harmful to people but noted that an animal study showed the chemical may alter hormone regulation and several other lab studies showed that bacteria may be able to evolve resistance to triclosan in a way that can help them also resist antibiotics." Whether it's safe or it's not, I always find some peace of mind by taking the natural road first. That's why I thought I'd share a few natural alternatives to antibacterial soaps, also an important part of first aid. Start out with the natural course, and it very rarely leads you to scary questions and breaking news later.

So what herbs are antibacterial? The list is seemingly endless, but some of the most common are: lavender (*Lavandula angustifolia*), rosemary (*Rosemarinus officinalis*), garlic, and peppermint (*Mentha piperita*). Apple cider vinegar is another natural item that provides antibacterial protection. Many of our herb friends are not only antibacterial but antifungal and antiviral as well. (Makes for a pretty good argument of natural versus manmade when you consider there's no hard evidence that the antibacterial soaps in question even work.) And according to the *Reference Guide to Essential Oils* by Connie and Alan Higley, all essential oils are antibacterial. Leaves you with quite a selection, doesn't it?

With the addition of a few drops, or a combination of any of these and other essential oils into a spray bottle of distilled water, you have a pretty fragrant antibacterial spray. I'd recommend using about a cup of water to 20 drops of oil. Experiment with blends that you like, and place them in a spray bottle. (Of course don't spray it in your eyes, eat it, or let your kids play with it. But you knew that already.)

A favorite of mine is Vinegar of the Four Thieves. This historical blend was said to protect four thieves from the Black Plague when they used it after robbing the dead bodies of plague victims. Gruesome story no doubt, and no one is certain of the validity of it all, but we do know the components of most Four Thieves recipes are pretty effective. There are literally dozens of variations to this recipe, but here's my own take, based on several I've seen:

Vinegar of the Four Thieves

4 Tbs. dried lavender
4 Tbs. dried rosemary
4 Tbs. dried wormwood
4 Tbs. dried mint (I use peppermint)
4 Tbs. dried sage
2 quarts apple cider vinegar

If you can crush up the herbs a bit with a mortar and pestle or run them through a coffee grinder reserved for your herbs, this will allow for better saturation. Place the herbs in a glass jar, pour the vinegar over it, and give it a vigorous shake. Put the jar in the sun for two or more weeks (I've read up to six weeks; this info varies). After two weeks, if you are so inclined, you can add a few cloves of garlic and let it sit for another week. I've seen recipes with and without garlic, but there are definitely antibacterial and antiviral benefits in adding it. I can also imagine the smell, so I'll leave this part up to you. I make mine without garlic so we can use it in public without chasing that public away. Strain the vinegar well and pour into spray bottles. You can carry it with you in a small bottle in your purse for when your kids have touched something icky or questionable, perhaps that shopping card handle.

Then of course there's always the old standby: Wash your hands thoroughly with regular soap. To get the benefits of herbs in there again, get soaps that contain essential oils.

If you're still worried about whether or not antibacterial soap is unsafe, natural alternatives are good to keep in mind. Remember, oftentimes if you start out with the natural solution, it doesn't really matter what the news says. What is called safe today might be called unsafe tomorrow, but that rarely happens in the herb world. Yes, there are herbs we need to be careful with, and the media often likes to squawk about them as well, but as in all of life, moderation is key. The good news is, plants seem to have a much better — and longer — track record for safe and effective use. I'm more than happy to stick with my botanical friends for my family's antibacterial concerns.

Remedies by Organ System

From your head to your toes, there are all sorts of things that can go awry with the body. Dealing with bodily discomforts is indeed a pain. They distract and for some they even depress. For people like us, looking to live a more healthy lifestyle, it adds the question, "How do I deal with this in the most natural way possible?" Thank goodness for the herbs once again. What follows is a compilation of remedies organized by organ system. While it's far from all-inclusive, it does cover a wide variety of the things so many of us deal with every day.

Cardiovascular Issues

I'm not talking the surefire way to reversing a heart attack here, but there are a few things that can be done to improve overall heart health through herbalism. Be sure, as with all herbal remedies, to let your doctor know what you're taking. If you're prone to heart problems, it would be even better to check with your doctor before adding any herbs to your routine. (Incidentally, if your doctor is totally opposed to adding any herbs or natural remedies to your medicinal repertoire, it may be time to find a doctor who is willing to work with you on a more natural approach. They are out there!)

High Blood Pressure

Taking medication for high blood pressure is something a lot of people would like to avoid. Side effects for these medications are often unpleasant and can result in a plethora of new issues. But it's also not healthy to avoid treating your high blood pressure. It's always a good idea to figure out what is causing it first. Is it your diet? Your lifestyle? Did your father, your grandfather, and various other relatives before you suffer from high blood pressure as well? Or maybe you're allergic to things like treadmills and gyms, and are much more comfortable relaxing on a couch most days.

If you're taking care of things like diet and exercise and you still suffer from high blood pressure, it may be time to try a few remedies from your herbal medicine chest. Again, tell your doctor anything you're planning on trying, especially if you're already taking blood pressure meds. Knowledge is definitely power when it comes to your health.

Perhaps you're the sort of person who worked a physical job your whole life. You were always on the go; the outdoors was your office and your arms and legs your high tech machinery. Nowadays, retirement has you sitting still a lot more than you prefer. After all, you can only rebuild the deck so many times before your wife gets frustrated and takes away the Home Depot card. So now, you're looking at a bit more sedentary life than you were once accustomed to, and your blood pressure isn't doing so hot. It's a little high, and the doc wants the numbers down. What do you do?

Possibly the most important herb for cardiovascular health is hawthorn (*Crataegus spp.*) It's especially great for the types of people described above, whose abruptly sedentary life has the blood pressure higher than healthy, but overall, this is a great herb for anyone looking to improve the blood pressure. A safe tonic, it can be taken daily. (**NOTE**: If you've been prescribed nitroglycerine to be taken regularly, don't take hawthorn unless you've checked with your physician and they give the okay.) For a tincture, try one made of berries and flowering branches, or just berries if that's all that's available to you. Ten to 30 drops up to 3 times a day can help overall heart health. If you prefer it as a tea, a cold infusion of the berries, taken 1 to 2 ounces twice a day makes for a delicious beverage that is mildly reminiscent of root beer or sassafras.

Combined with passionflower (*Passiflora incarnata*), you have a very nice herbal duo indeed. The passionflower allows you to relax, in particular if you're the sort of person who has a hard time unwinding if everything isn't under control. It's an arterial sedative that gets a high pulse down. A whole herb tincture is taken, 30 to 60 drops, up to four times a day. Although there is no drug-like effect, it is relaxing, so be sure to pay attention to how you react to it so you can tailor your dosage to your needs and your own constitution. Perhaps you won't want any in the morning, for instance.

Overall Heart Health

Again, I'll start right off with the hawthorn (*Crataegus spp.*) If you are concerned with your heart health for any reason, hawthorn is definitely the way to go. (**NOTE**: If you've been prescribed nitroglycerine to be taken regularly, don't take hawthorn unless you've checked with your physician and they give the okay. This bears repeating.) It's not something you grab if your left arm starts going numb or if you suddenly feel chest pain, but it is something to take over time and regularly to improve and strengthen. It dilates the coronary artery and moves blood through to the heart while strengthening and regulating the heartbeat. For people with degenerative heart disease or longtime smokers, people who suffer from a weak heart due to illness or infection, or arteriosclerosis, hawthorn's your herb. This is also great if you're the type who occasionally experiences a sort of skip in your heartbeat or an arrhythmic sensation that makes you stop and wonder "What on earth was that?"

Again, the dosage would be 10 to 30 drops up to 3 times a day for the flowering branch and berry tincture, or 1 to 2 ounces twice a day for the cold infusion of dried hawthorn berries.

41

If you're fortunate enough to have one of these thorny trees or shrubs near you, you can collect the berries in the fall and dry them yourself. This is one instance where any sort of hawthorn tree or shrub will do (as long as you're sure it's hawthorn), since there are so many subspecies even experts can't often tell one from the other! But one thing remains the same: the plant's amazing benefits to the heart.

Immortal (*Asclepias asperula*) is a sort of milkweed plant common in the Southwest. Taken regularly, 5 to 30 drops of the tincture up to 3 times a day, it's most helpful in slowing and strengthening the pulse in people who are otherwise healthy, active individuals but seem to be slow in getting the blood flowing in the morning. For an enlarged or weak heart, it's quite helpful.

Common milkweed (*Asclepias cornuta*), also known as pleurisy root, is a weaker form of the above, with more of a tonic-like effect. Also taken 5 to 30 drops up to 3 times a day, it's a less potent form if you're not in need of a strong medicine for more specific heart ailments.

You might also consider adding cayenne pepper (*Capsicum spp.*) to your daily repertoire for heart health. The people of Thailand aren't often prone to things like heart disease and arterial sclerosis due to their healthy consumption of hot peppers. I won't tell you to snack on the spicy little buggers, but I will tell you that taken as a tincture, you can reduce arterial plaque and fat deposits in the heart. A mere 5 to 15 drops of cayenne tincture in water taken up to 5 times a day is all that's needed to dilate those blood vessels, improve the health of your heart valves, and deliver aid to hypertension and viscous blood.

If you're concerned about the heat from the peppers, there's no need to worry. When taken in tincture form in water, the spiciness is no longer noticeable. And since the tincture is absorbed into the system before it reaches your intestinal tract, it's a safer way to go than to take cayenne in capsule form. Of course, if you do suffer from ulcers, this probably isn't your remedy. It also acts as a blood thinner, so be sure to tell your doctor you're taking it, or check first if you're already taking blood thinners or have plans for major surgery.

Digestive Issues

We've all suffered from digestive issues. Whether you're talking nausea due to nerves or diarrhea due to last night's trip to Bob's Wet Burrito Bar, it's good to have a handle on several natural remedies so you know what to do when your stomach starts talking - and you don't like what it's saying.

Diarrhea, Vomiting, and Nausea

Whether your child comes home from school with an upset tummy, a case of "the runs," or often more unpleasantly, vomiting, it's good to have a few natural remedies at the ready. There are a lot of different ways to settle the upset tummy and quell diarrhea and vomiting with herbs, but I like this one because it's simple and involves an ingredient most of us have in the home all the time. It's a basic rice tea.

To prepare rice tea, boil ½ cup of rice (regular, not instant) in about 6 cups of water for 15 minutes. Strain out the rice. You can flavor the tea with a dash of vanilla extract if you wish, and perhaps a dash of cinnamon. Serve it up warm. Perhaps you'll find you enjoy drinking the tea just for pleasure.

Peppermint tea is another excellent choice, and most people enjoy this safe and delicious remedy. Taken as needed, a cup of the tea is antimicrobial and antiviral, and can often relieve symptoms of diarrhea, vomiting, or nausea quickly.

One thing I think is important to point out here: If there is vomiting or diarrhea, you may not want to stop it immediately. Our first reaction, especially as parents, is to put an end to the discomfort, and quickly. But if your child (or you) has eaten something bad, for instance, the body's natural defense is to toss it out whether through one end or the other. Unpleasant? Yes, but necessary. Consider allowing for a few "cookie tosses" before serving the tea. Of course, that may occur anyway, while you're waiting for the tea to boil. After the body has purged, it's nice to settle things down and restore some strength.

Cardamom (*Elettaria cardamomum*) is a wonderful herb probably most recognizable to us in the West as a fragrant Indian cooking spice. But what this plant's lovely little seedpods hold is much more than culinary delight. Its use as one of the more tasty natural remedies for nausea and the queasy stomach sets it apart.

Cardamom is actually a member of the ginger family. As you may already know, ginger is also a useful anti-nausea remedy, but what's so charming about cardamom is its tidy packaging in the form of a pod, making it nature's portable solution for the queasies.

The pods keep well for years. I have a batch of pods that I use that was purchased about four or five years ago, and they're still very much effective.

To use a cardamom pod to ease stomach upset, break open the outside and remove the small black seeds. You can break off a seed (they're sort of segmented chunks) and suck on the small piece, occasionally crunching it a bit with your teeth. You can swallow it when you're done if you wish, or spit it out; it's up to you. Or try a tincture, 5 to 10 drops in some water as needed. But the seeds are more fun.

You'll find the cardamom tastes so good and refreshing that you may enjoy carrying a few in your purse or pocket to use as breath fresheners. You'll also find cardamom such an impressive natural remedy for general queasiness, morning sickness, even a nervous stomach, that you'll want to keep them as a permanent member of your herbal medicine cabinet.

Acid Indigestion

Instead of reaching for that unnaturally pink goop in a bottle, there are a few wonderful herbs just waiting to come to your rescue. When indigestion strikes, you can give the following teas a try: fennel (*Foeniculum vulgare*), catmint (*Nepeta cataria*), chamomile (*Matricaria recutita*), or peppermint (*Mentha piperita*). There are literally so many to choose from for acid indigestion that I wouldn't bother to list them all here. But these are a few easy ones to find. If you'd like to go with fennel, no need to rush out for fennel tea bags. Don't forget that it's okay to snag stuff out of your spice cupboard too. Of course, if you want to build up an herbal medicine cabinet, it's cheaper to buy something like fennel from your local health food store in bulk. Those tiny overpriced bottles of cooking spices at the supermarket are not only way too expensive — they've sometimes been sitting there too long to do much anymore. But they do work in a pinch.

Bloating

If you're feeling bloated, or if your fingers are starting to look like little Vienna sausages due to some nasty water retention, consider forgoing the water pills. They'll drain much more than just water from your system. With it goes much needed potassium, not to mention a whole host of other essentials your body needs. Instead, consider the lovely dandelion plant (*Taraxacum officinale*). This amazing powerhouse of vitamins and minerals performs a sort of magic trick when it comes to ridding the bloat. You see, dandelion is full of potassium. And it's a great diuretic. Somehow, it manages to keep your body in balance — releasing excess water and maintaining healthy levels of potassium. Something your average water pill is unable to accomplish.

To enjoy the benefits of dandelion for water retention relief, you can either tincture the whole plant — flower, stem, leaves and all (spring plants are best) — or purchase a quality fresh whole plant tincture. Take 30 to 60 drops up to 4 times a day. And don't forget to drink more water. While this may seem counterintuitive, the more water you drink, the more freely your body is able to flush your system. Since most Americans are actually walking around dehydrated, their bodies hang onto every bit of water they can, often causing bloating and discomfort. Drink more water, lose more water. Simple as that.

Gastroesophageal Reflux Disease (GERD)

Gastroesophageal reflux disease (GERD) is a "condition in which acid, bile and partially-digested food in the stomach back up into the esophagus." For many people, this all too common ailment is making a difficult time of their daily lives. First, try not to eat when you're stressed. So many of us eat in a hurry, under pressure, or when we're completely frazzled — as if we're still those cave men and women trying to get a quick meal in before the saber tooth comes along to claim his portion. Before eating, give yourself a few moments of peace and quiet. During meals, chew thoroughly to aid in digestion. And think of Uncle Howard, the guy who always loosened his belt at the dinner table: Don't wear clothing that restricts your stomach. (And here you thought Uncle Howard was just a little gross.)

Try and wait three hours after eating before lying down. And when you do tuck in for the night, try sleeping on your left side, which will keep your stomach below your esophagus.

That most versatile of herbal remedies, chamomile (*Matricaria recutita*), produces a fabulous tea that is known for its ability to soothe gastrointestinal spasms, so a cup of this warm herbal brew may be just the thing to naturally relax your GERD.

It's always good to consult your doctor, but by trying a few natural remedies before taking the trip to the office, conditions like GERD are sometimes controllable without the need for pharmaceuticals. Nature's just smart that way. And so is Uncle Howard.

Hemorrhoids

We've all seen the commercials of squirming people making awful faces and dancing around in their seats while in public. Maybe we've even been those people from time to time. But there's no need to slather on the chemicals to cure the situation. Instead, try some witch hazel (*Hamamelis*), which soothes and tones varicose veins and other skin problems. It's a mild astringent usually made from the bark of the witch hazel tree, and it's readily available at pharmacies and health food stores.

Or, if you have access to a witch hazel tree or shrub, you can make your own. Although the bark is generally the part of the plant used, you might want to see how the leaves work for you. Well-known herbalist Samuel Thomson (1769 - 1843) used the leaves quite successfully.

If your hemorrhoids start bleeding, some shepherd's purse (*Capsella bursa-pastoris*) can fix you in a flash. Apply the cool tea topically for relief. Alternately, if the bleeding hemorrhoids are more of a long-term oozing problem, consider adding cinnamon to your diet. Sprinkle it on your oatmeal, your toast, and whatever else floats your boat. You may just lower your cholesterol and blood sugar while you're at it.

When hemorrhoids are a persistent problem, you'll definitely need to consider your diet, ensuring there's enough fiber intake. Take a look at how often you're emptying your bowels as well. That's vitally important; not going once a day or more is a bad sign and can be the cause of your hemorrhoids. See the following section on constipation if you're having trouble.

Constipation

Closely related to the hemorrhoid issue, this section could count as Hemorrhoids Part 2. Treating constipation and making sure you're regular is key in ending the discomfort of hemorrhoids, not to mention ridding your body of a whole host of other health concerns. Being a crankypants isn't the only side effect. Less energy, sluggishness, bloating, and discomfort are just a few more. Finding healthy ways to aid in digestion is extremely important for your entire constitution, and fortunately, there are many ways you can deal with this.

Sunflower seeds are one tasty way to help you out of a tight spot. The oils of the seeds are lubricating, and the seeds themselves both stimulate bile and offer the body the fiber it needs.

A similar choice is flax seed, which can be eaten as they are. They taste mildly of walnuts, and must be chewed — or freshly ground — for best effect. If you're not very excited about munching away at 1 or 2 teaspoons of these each day, you can sprinkle ground flax seed on just about anything you like; from oatmeal to rice to salads. Just make sure to get it added to your diet. They're loaded with omega-3's and can and should be eaten daily to maintain regularity. You'll even find your hair and skin become healthier and shinier after a couple of months of usage, too. There are numerous benefits to flax, and anyone would do well to incorporate them as a regular part of their diet. But do indeed try and buy the seeds whole, then chew them well or grind right before use. This will allow you to get the most benefit from these tiny but powerful seeds.

Slippery elm bark (*Ulmus rubra*) is another option. Prepared as a gruel, you can even flavor it with a bit of maple syrup or honey. This is a nice one for kids, who often enjoy the warm breakfast-like approach to relieving their symptoms. To make the gruel, mix 1 ½ tsp. slippery elm bark powder with ¼ cup of water in a pan, and stir well to make a paste. Stirring constantly, slowly pour in 1 ½ to 2 cups of boiling water, and continue to stir it for another 2 minutes with a whisk or a spoon. At this point, flavor it with whatever you enjoy eating in oatmeal: raisins, honey, cinnamon, dates, walnuts, etc. 1 to 2 cups of this gruel eaten 1 to 3 times a day should restore law and order soon.

Senna (*Cassia marilandica*) is a popular choice for constipation. For hemorrhoids, piles, and rectal fissures, you need to take things easy on the tissues. Taking senna won't irritate injuries to the descending colon, either. It's mildly tonic to the digestive system. A tea made of senna leaves taken at bedtime will help move the bowels by morning. Even more effective than the senna leaves are the pods. Placing 10 to 15 senna pods in water for ½ hour before drinking, pods and all, is an excellent way to restore order when your bowels aren't living up to their end of the bargain. However, senna isn't for everyday use, and oftentimes people rely on it until they can't go without it. Use it to get yourself back on track if needed, but not daily to keep yourself regular. Flax seed can do that.

Halitosis

Oh, the embarrassment! You didn't mean to eat a bag of garlic breadsticks and an anchovy onion salad, but you've gone and done it anyway, and now you just got a last-minute urge to go to the movies. Since your local theater doesn't offer private box seats with heavy curtains, and since you'd probably get kicked out if you tried to get through the doors sporting a bandanna stretched across the lower half of your face, what do you do now? All the toothpaste in the world isn't gonna cure this.

Not to worry, my friend. Keep a few of these remedies — even in your pocket — for just such emergencies.

Cardamom pods (*Elettaria cardamomum*) are an excellent breath remedy. They smell fantastic, they taste great, and they're entirely portable, coming in their own naturally grown wrappers. Keep a tin of the pods in their entirety in your purse or the glove compartment of your car; wherever you need some refreshment in a pinch. Simply break open a pod and pull out one or two of the tiny black segments inside. (You'll notice the interior contains long strips of black seeds that are easily broken into little pebbly pieces.) Suck on the cardamom for as long as you need. You can either spit it out when you're done or chew it up and swallow it. And if that dinner out with friends ever gives you a bout of nausea, you can grab for the cardamom too. It's perfect for the queasies caused by anything from too many curly fries to finding out your mother-in-law is paying you a surprise visit. In five minutes.

Other simple breath-freshening herbs that can easily tag along with you are black peppercorns and cloves. The peppercorns are surprisingly tasty and refreshing, and if you enjoy the taste of cloves, you can keep one of those babies in your mouth for a long time without it losing its potency.

If you're out to dinner and you're lucky enough to have an old-fashioned curly parsley garnish on the side, don't leave it behind. Munch on it. Maybe don't be all obvious about the fact that you're relishing your garnish, but that dose of parsley will help neutralize your dinner and make it possible for you to enjoy the rest of your evening without offending your companions.

Urinary Tract Infections

If there's one thing sure to turn life upside down for awhile, it's a urinary tract infection, or UTI. A UTI is a bacterial infection in the bladder or kidneys. If it's in your bladder, you'll probably feel like you have to pee a lot, even when you don't really have to. You might be getting up several times in the night, and you're probably feeling some pain and discomfort, sometimes a burning sensation in the area above your pubic bone. A bad infection may come with blood in the urine and a fever, so if this happens, get to a doctor! That's also the case if you're thinking it's a kidney infection, which includes back pain, oftentimes vomiting, and high spiky fevers. Natural remedies are great, but when you're getting things like bleeding, fevers, and vomiting, it's best to avoid self-treatment. But if you're pretty sure you're at the beginning stages, there are natural remedies to help you get rid of a urinary tract infection. And this one is simple for any age: asparagus.

Asparagus spears, fresh or frozen, are a great way to douse the flames of UTI's for adults and children alike. If you have an infection, your pee probably already smells a little off, anyway, and asparagus is sure to add a new layer to this. But it's fantastic for the urinary tract. You don't have to scarf it down plain, either. You can steam it, bake it – I've even had it grilled, which is fantastic. A soup is a nice way to go because you're not dumping out the vitamin-rich water it cooks in. It's also great in a stir fry with a little elephant garlic and kale, two other extremely healthy foods that'd be good to have on your side about now.

If your kids aren't hip to asparagus, you could try the stir fry with small pieces of asparagus tucked in, mixed with some of their more favorite vegetables so maybe they won't notice what you're up to.

Cranberry juice is probably the most common natural remedy discussed for UTI's. Even the doctors recognize this one. Cranberry juice is a great remedy for bladder infections, but if you're pulling the first juice you find off the grocery store shelf, you might be feeding that infection instead. Almost every commercial cranberry juice I've ever looked at contains added sugars and/or high fructose corn syrup. Infections love a good dose of sugar. For them, it's dinner in a nice restaurant. So do yourself a big favor and get some pure juice from a health food store. Or better yet, purchase a bag or two of fresh cranberries when you can. Cook them according to package instructions and avoid the sugar. I know, I know. Sour, isn't it? But it works and it's naturally good.

If you're prone to UTI's, purchase bags of fresh cranberry in the fall and toss them into the freezer for later. They freeze whole very well.

Another fantastic solution is acidophilus. Acidophilus works for all kinds of infections, including sinus, yeast, bronchial, ear... you name it. The trick here is to make sure you're getting a good quality acidophilus, and look for one that needs refrigeration. Also make sure to check the expiration date. Acidophilus is a live culture, so you don't want to pay for expired product. Take the pills according to the package instructions, and just like an antibiotic, try hard not to miss a dose.

For prevention, women may discover their soap choice will make a drastic difference. Oftentimes women prone to bladder infections will, in desperation, use a lot of harsh soap to cleanse where they think bacteria is entering. Turns out all that soap is causing the infections to return again and again. After switching to a natural vegetable glycerin soap, many women completely end their cycle of UTI's. There are lots of glycerin soaps out there, and many of them get fancy and scented. Try to get the most pure vegetable glycerin soap you can, without all the additives. It's even great on baby fine hair as an alternative to baby shampoos, and there are no nasty chemicals. A word of warning: I once bought plain vegetable glycerin thinking I was getting a great deal on a big bottle of it. If it doesn't mention the word "soap," it's not going to have the same cleansing effect, so make sure you get the right thing.

If you've got access to fresh cleavers (*Galium aparine*) during spring and summer months, you can run them through a juicer and drink the juice. Or find a fresh plant tincture, 1 to 2 teaspoons taken up to 4 times daily. You can also go with dried cleavers and prepare a tea. Either way you choose, partake of your cleavers 3 times a day until your infection is gone. Cleavers also relieves painful urination and can rid you of water retention and edema. It's also helpful for people who have a tendency towards kidney stones, but I wouldn't go with dried cleavers for tea in this case. Fresh forms are best.

I recently found a huge stand of pipsissewa (*Chimaphila*) during a walk in the woods. The plant was gorgeous and delicate. I didn't pick any but decided to enjoy the sight of all those lovely little forest blooms. I don't see pipsissewa out in the wild often where I live, and perhaps you don't either. But it is a plant you can get in herbal commerce if not on the forest floor, so if you're prone to bladder infections, keep an eye out for this beauty. It's a good choice if you have burning, a strong urge to urinate, and you get very little for your efforts - and what you do get is cloudy. You can purchase it dried for tea or as a tincture. For tea, drink 4 to 8 ounces 4 times a day. Tincture, try 20 to 50 drops in a little water 4 times a day. Pipsissewa is one more herb that can benefit those who are prone to kidney stones when used regularly as a preventive measure.

Always remember: Natural remedies such as asparagus or cleavers that are used to relieve urinary tract infections are great to know, especially as part of a parent's health care arsenal. But watch things closely with something like bladder and kidney infections. Yes, avoiding a trip to the doctor and a round of antibiotics is possible, but if things turn more serious with fevers, vomiting, blood in the urine, or pain that just doesn't seem right, see your doctor right away.

PMS

Got cramps? How about bloating up like a blowfish, enough irritability to scare a WWF professional wrestler, flow as heavy as Niagara? Then I certainly don't blame you for being cranky. When that menstrual monster rears its ugly head and makes it impossible for you to remember what "normal" is, there are some natural period remedies to keep at your side so you don't break any more dishes.

First things first: Get some dried raspberry leaf (*Rubus idaeus*). This makes a delicious tea that covers a wide range of symptoms, including cramping, bloating, and irregular bleeding. You can drink several cups of it a day (as much as needed), and it's pretty good stuff, in my opinion. A little honey and your day may start getting sweeter again.

If your period is unusually heavy, you can try some yarrow. Yes, yarrow is an herb that's famous for its ability to stop wounds from bleeding, but interestingly enough, it works internally as well. No, it won't stop your period altogether (drat), but it will regulate excessive and heavy menstrual cycles. In fact, if you have a very light period and need it to kick into gear, yarrow will assist you with that as well. You can make a tea out of the dried flowering tops, or you can take it as a tincture. In this instance I think the tea works a bit better, however. For intensely heavy flow, I recommend even trying both. Take the tincture immediately while you wait for your tea to steep.

For natural pain relief, ginger tea is another favorite. It helps take the edge off the cramping, and it's soothing as well, but it can increase your flow, so if that's already an issue for you, you might try some valerian instead.

If you're extra edgy and unable to sleep, and if you've got cramps to top it all off, valerian (*Valeriana officinalis*) is very helpful. As a tea, take 4 to 6 ounces; tincture, 30 to 90 drops. Yes, it smells like cat pee. But it works incredibly well. It's so relaxing that you shouldn't drink valerian tea and drive. No heavy machinery, no choosing that day to go to battle, etc. And don't take it for days at a time, or you may start to feel depressed and unmotivated. Take it when you need it, and stop taking it when you don't.

Motherwort. It just sounds comforting, doesn't it? This famous women's herb is antispasmodic, sedative, regulates your flow, and is great when menses is delayed due to stress. Anxiety, tension, and irregular flow all go bye-bye with motherwort (*Leonurus cardiaca*). And when you're just plain stressed and anxious, enduring a racing heart and that "I want my mommy" sensation even the most independent of adults occasionally experience, motherwort is perfect for you. It's safe and mild and is suited to daily use as a healthful tonic for women's issues, heart health, and emotional instability. You can take 30 to 60 drops of the tincture up to 4 times a day, or 2 to 4 ounces of the tea up to 4 times a day.

My 5-year-old son said it best one day when he asked me if I knew what motherwort was used for. "What?" I asked. He replied, "It's for when you need your mommy but she's not there. You take motherwort and it feels like she's with you." Well said, young grasshopper. Well said.

Respiratory Problems

If you're interested in treating allergies, asthma, and other respiratory ailments with herbs and natural remedies, the possibilities are endless. As with most of herbal medicine, the results largely depend on what is causing your symptoms and what kinds of allergies and asthma you suffer from. What follows here are a few of my favorite remedies, most of which I've actually tested on myself. I've left out the ones that resulted in hallucinations and visions of singing angels.

I might admit to a lack of visions during experimentation, but I can tell you that the ones included here are the safest I know of. And they've worked for me and for others who I've shared them with.

Allergies

Oddly enough, one great allergy herb may be a plant you've been blaming for your symptoms to begin with. Goldenrod (*Solidago spp.*) is often accused of causing sniffling and sneezing when it's in bloom. However, the goldenrod plant requires pollination by insects because its pollen is just too darned heavy for the wind to do the job – which means there's really not a bunch of Goldenrod pollen floating around. True, many people are allergic when coming into contact, but much of the time what you're reacting to is probably the ragweed which grows in the same areas as the goldenrod. But since ragweed has green and rather indiscriminate flowers, the flashy goldenrod gets noticed and takes the blame instead.

Goldenrod is the one to choose when your allergies give you a runny nose or postnasal drip with a tickly cough. Tincture is the best way to go with this one. You can tincture the flowering tops yourself, if you don't mind braving the fields of that sneaky ragweed hiding behind it. Take 30 to 40 drops of the tincture up to 5 times a day.

If you're really brave (or if you've got one of those friends for whom allergies are not an issue), you can tincture the ragweed too (*Ambrosia*). As crazy as it sounds, ragweed makes for a great hay fever and allergy tincture of its own. You can tincture the leaves or buy ragweed leaf tincture already prepared, and take 20 to 40 drops up to 4 times a day, for relief from your allergies and hay fever.

Asthma

If asthma gives you a chronic and persistent cough that makes your lungs feel all gooped up, elecampane (*Inula helenium*) is a good expectorant. It's also good for general lung health, as it improves the mucus membrane. Use this one as a tea, a strong decoction at 2 to 6 ounces taken up to 3 times a day. Dried root cut for tea makes for a must-have remedy for the heavy, full lungs of many asthmatics. It has an aromatic woody smell that at first sniff may have you turning up your nose. Second sniff? You'll like it. It's definitely a strong, camphor-like herb, and upon giving it a whiff, you'll know why it works as well as it does. Alternatively, tincture is fine. Take 10 to 30 drops up to 4 times a day.

Another benefit to elecampane: It improves the appetite. Anyone who's ever experienced breathing difficulties knows that the last thing you feel like doing is eating. Maybe it's the gulping of air, or perhaps it has more to do with the psychological aspect of filling your mouth with anything but oxygen. Either way, elecampane gives you ease of breathing and stimulates the appetite, making you feel more like yourself again. It doesn't hurt that it tends to give one a general sense of wellbeing too.

One excellent remedy for any lung ailment (asthma in particular) is white pine bark (*Pinus strobus*). When lungs feel full and tight, white pine opens things up, and in a hurry. You can take 6 to 8 ounces of the tea whenever you feel you need it. It's wise to store up as much of this as you can; the nice part is you can harvest it anytime of year. I often go into the woods in late spring, but I've gone year round and still had great results with it. You can purchase the bark, or you can find a nice white pine tree in a clean, unpolluted area. Trim the ends of the branches off; no exact science here. The smaller ones are practical because they're easier to deal with, and peeling the bark off the larger branches for drying is no easy task. With the small ones, you can just yank off all the needles and cut up the whole branch in small pieces, then spread them out to dry. Larger branches require you to strip off the bark with a knife, then cut up the bark before drying. An Eastern European friend of mine says that back in the Old Country, they like spring's new growth best.

Store the dried white pine in a clean dry jar out of direct sunlight, and use about a teaspoonful in a cup of boiling water. Cover to steep so the volatile oils don't escape. After about 20 to 30 minutes (if you can wait that long), strain and sip. It's a bit sticky on the lips, I know, but it works fast. It clears things up within 20 to 30 minutes, and you'll usually feel back to normal once again.

When you've been suffering from asthma over a few day's time and your lungs feel tighter and tighter, they are most likely filled with old mucus that needs to come out. In this instance, try mullein leaf tea or tincture. Mullein (*Verbascum thapsis*) is a common herb that grows in wasteland areas, gravelly spots, and places other plants fear not tread. If you know the plant and want to harvest it yourself, that's great. Just be careful where you pick it because it likes to grow in depressed, abused areas that may not produce plants healthy for human consumption. Old busted up parking lots, for instance, aren't your best bet. You can buy mullein leaf in tea bags, and some people prefer that. Mullein has little bitty hairs growing on the mature leaves that can irritate the throat and feel unpleasant, and commercially prepared mullein seems to be void of those. As with any commercially prepared herb, make sure it hasn't been sitting on the shelf for years. Herbs lose their potency over time, and the fresher the better. Always.

You can also opt to go with the tincture instead. Use 30 to 90 drops in water, waiting maybe 20 to 30 minutes before taking another dose if needed. It's a pretty safe herb, so if you need more than one or two rounds, you can. But beware that it's going to move the congestion out of the lungs through coughing, so make sure you wait in between dosages a full 20 to 30 minutes. In my own haste to breathe, I've taken several heavy shots of mullein leaf tincture in a row, giving me such a bout of coughing that, while it did clear out my lungs and bring me relief, the coughing fits were enough to wear me out for the rest of the day. Give it the time it needs to work and it will, without ringing you out like a used dishrag.

You can take mullein tincture daily as a safe and healthy tonic. It improves lung function and can aid in overall asthma relief if taken over a period of time. Twenty to 40 drops in some water up to 3 times daily is a good place to start. It's completely safe to take on a regular basis, so stock up, all ye who suffer from asthma!

Bronchitis

I first discussed the following onion remedy on a blog of mine, www.dkMommySpot.com. One wonderful 70-year-old reader from Illinois said her mother and grandmother always used onions on her and her siblings for their lung issues. She still relies on onions as her first defense against lung ailments. The smell of this remedy may make everyone hungry, but it's sure to help break up the lung congestion from the bronchitis. Fry up some onions and let them cool until they're not too hot to handle. Rub the bronchitis sufferer's chest with olive oil, then lay the onions on the chest. Cover the onions with a thick cloth, preferably an old cotton towel or a piece of flannel. Use a hot water bottle to place over the towel; please be extra careful with the heat, especially with young children. This remedy requires your constant supervision with the young ones.

When you're done, your patient will smell a bit like dinner, but the whole family will be breathing easier knowing relief has been found.

Common milkweed (Asclepias cornuta), also known as pleurisy root, is a nice mild expectorant that many find to be helpful during bouts of bronchitis. It's also a good thing to keep around for the initial stages of a chest cold. Five to 30 drops of the tincture can be taken up to 3 times a day for relief.

If you've been suffering from bronchitis for awhile and you're too darned tired to cough anymore, start on some osha (*Ligusticum porteri*). It's just right for a dry and irritated cough and will aid in getting the last of that junk out of your chest when it doesn't want to move. When taken as either tea or tincture, it leaves your system through your exhalations, putting an end to bacteria and viruses sitting in your lungs as it passes through. For the tincture, take 20 to 60 drops up to 3 times daily; but if your symptoms are more severe, you can take 60 to 120 drops every 2 hours until the symptoms subside. With the lower dosage, it will often take a day or two to start to work, but work it will. It's also helpful with upper respiratory infections and is a nice herb to add to echinacea, as the two together will heighten your immune system.

Dry Lungs

For a lovely and delicious tea that helps soothe dry and irritated lungs, try hibiscus (*Hibiscus sabdariffa*). It not only improves the mucous secretion, it's also an immunostimulant which increases the macrophages in your system, healthy infection-eating fellows who will gobble up pathogens and cellular debris like your family goes after Thanksgiving turkey.

Balsamroot (*Balsamorhiza*) brings moisture to dry bronchi and is another immunostimulant; it's similar to echinacea. The tea is a little bitter, so if you don't care for it, you can try the tincture taken 20 to 50 drops in hot water up to 4 times a day.

Muscles & Joints

Sometimes it's temporary — a little too much strain on the back while attempting a Wonder Woman lift. Other times it's a more permanently painful situation, such as arthritis. No two ways about it, muscle and joint pain is no picnic. Figuring out how to put an end to it is always welcome knowledge, and with a few herbs at your side, pain free days may be a few good cups of tea away.

Sore Muscles

Whether the kids' muscles ache from a day of lugging all those schoolbooks and partaking in extra hard play, or you're just plain worn out after yet another Monday, it's good to have some muscle liniment. It's so easy to make your own that purchasing it won't cross your mind after making that first batch.

This liniment recipe is a hot one, and it takes nothing more than what you probably already have in the kitchen cupboards. Take 1 teaspoon of dried cayenne pepper powder (*Capsicum*) and add it to 2 ounces of olive oil. I use a little egg whisker to blend it all together. If you're able to let it sit for at least a few days, it'll work better, but if you're aching to use it right away, that's okay too. Just make sure it's well blended. That's it. Now you're ready to rub away the aches and pains. (Please wash your hands thoroughly after usage, and don't touch your eyes. Also, keep it out of reach of children.)

This next remedy is also an easy one, but you must make it ahead of time and keep it on hand. Take one tablespoon of powdered goldenseal (*Hydrastis canadensis*), and mix it with one cup of vodka (the cheap kind works fine, and you'll be less tempted to just drink it instead.) Let it sit for two weeks. You can shake it every now and then or not; usually the alcohol does all the work for you, anyway. After two weeks, you can rub it on sore muscles with a cotton ball to ease the pain.

Now go forth and do strenuous things without fear. Ride that bike. Run through the sprinkler. Learn downward facing dog. For tomorrow, when the sore muscles remind you that you are not five years old (what were you thinking, out there on that skateboard?), you have the natural remedy for healing those aching muscles.

Musculoskeletal Injuries

Broken bones, bad knee joints, tendonitis, torn rotator cuffs, spinal and disc injuries, arthritis, torn ligaments, etc. I could write a separate section for each of these, but I'd only have to repeat it over and over again: solomon's seal, solomon's seal, solomon's seal (*Polygonatum multiflorum, Polygonatum multiflorum, Polygonatum multiflorum*). I make a tincture of the root of this plant, and everyone I know who has ever tried it checks in with me regularly to see if I've got the new batch ready yet. Fortunately, I've got one heck of a place for responsible wildcrafting of this amazing plant. No one seems to really know how this plant works, but the key here is that it does. Applied topically as a tincture, solomon's seal (or false solomon's seal [*Smilacina racemosa*], which works just the same) has almost immediate results. I've tested this several times over, and on varying unsuspecting people. The first time I ever used it, I felt the pain leave almost immediately. I thought it was the mind playing tricks on me. "Sure," thought I, "Fabulous herbalist you are. Falling for the power of suggestion like that." Scoff, scoff. But when I passed some on to my parents, my dad called me up about five minutes after his first go at the stuff. "I don't hurt! How come I don't hurt? I just put this stuff on!" Every time I give the tincture to someone, I purposely "forget" to tell them about the immediate pain relieving factor. Then they call me.

Unfortunately, this isn't one of those things that relieves pain every day for the rest of your life. And it's not going to work if you have plain old sore muscles or a headache or a stubbed toe, etc. This is a ligament and joint specialist. It does, however, have the ability to help heal the tears and strains we put those ligaments, tendons, and joints under. Over time with consistent usage, it'll help you heal faster; some herbalists even use this with broken bones, and with real results.

You don't need much of the tincture to see results. Just 5 to 10 drops, sometimes less, placed on the area and massaged in, whenever you feel you need it.

If you'd like to make it yourself, you can even grow solomon's seal in your own garden. I've seen this plant in our local gardening center in the native plants section (I'm in Michigan), so ask around. You'll want to plant several of them if you've got your own medicinal herb garden. Each year the root grows longer, and you can remove the tail end of the root, leaving a few "knuckles" of the root attached to the plant so it continues to grow. It takes a little trickery to get the root out without destroying the whole plant, but you follow the root along in the dirt with your fingers, bypassing a few inches before digging up the tail end. Since the root grows horizontally, perhaps 3 to 5 inches underground, and not straight down into the dirt, you can indeed follow it along pretty easily after a few tries.

My best anecdote with this plant? I'd told my friend about its ability to heal, and later went on to tell her how my poor dog has such bad hips and always has. She said, "Why don't you use that solomon's seal?" I did the proper head slap, then next time my dog's hips froze up, I placed a few drops on his hindquarters and rubbed it in. I was amazed at the results. Ever since that day, he backs up to me as soon as he sees his dropper bottle, waiting for his solomon's seal. As long as he's got his tincture, stairs are a breeze for him. And he doesn't suffer from the power of suggestion, either. Good dog.

Carpal Tunnel Syndrome

Typing, waiting tables, handiwork of all sorts – carpal tunnel syndrome is a painful problem for many. While more severe cases may require surgery, for the less severe case there are several natural remedies that can relieve the symptoms of carpal tunnel syndrome.

Take, for instance, ginger. 300 mg. taken twice a day, or taken as a tea, can help ease the pains of carpal tunnel. Turmeric (*Curcuma longa*) is another excellent anti-inflammatory, backed by much research around the world. I prefer it as a tincture, 30 to 40 drops taken 2 to 5 times a day, but capsules are also available. Flaxseed oil is a helpful aid as well. You can either add ground flaxseed to your diet (a teaspoon or two a day sprinkled on food, in beverages, etc.) or take it in a liquid capsule at about 2,000 mg. daily.

A simple thing such as drinking plenty of water can help too. Rehydrating the entire body and getting things moving can be an effective pain reducer. So can exercise and movement. Take time from your typing, physical strains, and other pain-causing activities to stretch and flex the wrists and hands. It will help circulate the blood and loosen tightness.

Hand and arm massaging is also of benefit. I like to use the cayenne pepper liniment discussed in the "Sore Muscles" section to massage on the skin. While you have to make sure to wash hands thoroughly after use (not fun in the eyes), the cayenne reduces pain quite well.

If pain persists, visit your doctor. But for many people these few simple natural remedies will work wonders for reducing the pain of carpal tunnel syndrome.

Arthritis

Unfortunately, arthritis isn't just for grandma anymore. An increasing number of us experience this painful and sometimes debilitating condition, but nature abounds with botanical relief.

Turmeric (*Curcuma longa*), as mentioned previously, is one fantastic anti-inflammatory and can bring serious relief to all sorts of aches and pains due to inflamed conditions. While this isn't something one should take if one has gallstones, the pain relieving effects cannot be denied or overlooked. Thirty to 40 drops of tincture taken 2 to 5 times a day can be quite a help when you're going through a serious bout of arthritis.

Many people have opted for the relief brought on by capsacin creams, and this is an instance when one purchased from a pharmacy or health food store is probably your best bet, although some people do make their own. These creams work by stimulating the nerves in aching areas and is especially helpful for people with rheumatoid arthritis. The first day of using a capsacin cream can be an uncomfortable experience as the cream goes to work literally exhausting the nerve endings. After a period of two to three days, the pain begins to be relieved, and a numbing sensation replaces pain upon application. This process is called "counter irritation." So if you're willing to get through the initial discomfort, this is a good remedy that will have effect for a long while.

Depression, Anxiety, Insomnia

Nothing can stop life in its tracks quite like depression, anxiety, or other mental illnesses. While serious bouts definitely require the attention of professionals such as doctors and counselors who can help get you through the pain and disruption, even the downright misery, herbs can often give you a hand up before things get too serious. And let's face it, we all find ourselves going through rough patches from time to time. But if things are truly serious, it is vitally important to get help. Go tell a friend. If you don't have a friend you feel comfortable sharing with, find a counselor or a hotline; a sympathetic and impartial ear that can hear you out and head you towards recovery. If you haven't gotten to that point yet but feel you're starting the spiral downward, here are a few of the many herbs I'd recommend.

Depression

There are so many herbs that seem to specialize in depression that I can only offer up a few here. But I've chosen the ones that are considered most effective by herbalists and are, for the most part, easiest to get a hold of.

I'm starting with the obvious because it truly is an antidepression wonder. St. John's-wort (*Hypericum perforatum*) may sound almost cliche these days when discussing the natural antidepresssant, but there's a very good reason its name surfaces again and again. It works. I know, I know. You've heard conflicting reports on the news, and oddly, medical studies funded by major pharmaceutical companies keep coming up with negative findings on our herb friends (interesting, when you consider most modern pharmaceuticals have stemmed from a plant, a tree, a tiny flower, albeit a twisted and rewired version of the original.) And of the herb friends, St. John's-wort is certainly worthy of mention here. This is especially helpful for people who have a depression that seems to be mixed with anger. If you've got the "yo-yo" type up and down depression with bouts of anger, St. John's-wort is for you. It also works well for seasonal depression and for occasional bouts of sadness that appears to have no explanation. Twenty to 30 drops, up to 3 times a day, of the fresh flowering plant tincture is a good way to start. (Taken before bed, it may make you a bit too awake, so beware.) I'd suggest starting on the low side and working your way up until you find the dosage that works for you. While this can bring some relief after the very first dosage, a more pronounced difference can be felt over time. Take caution, however: St. John's-wort does make people more prone to photosensitivity, so be careful if spending long periods of time in the sun or near ultraviolet rays. Also, be sure to tell your doctor you're taking it. If you're already on an antidepressant, for instance, you don't want to include any herbs until you know if they'll interfere with your current meds. St. John's-wort does indeed work as a reuptake inhibitor, much the same as many prescription meds for depression.

Wild oat (*Avena sativa*) offers relief for many almost instantly. If you've found yourself staring down into a hole that you can't seem to pull out of, wild oat can be an important remedy for you. Take 10 to 20 drops of fresh plant tincture, up to 4 times a day; or if you prefer tea, use the wild oat straw — dried but green in color — and drink 4 to 8 ounces, up to 4 times a day.

If you're feeling as if your only identity these days is your depression, try some anemone (*Anemone hirsutissima*), otherwise known as pasque flower, before reaching for the antidepressants. This is also good for people who feel their grief has moved in to stay, or if the depression brings physical pain like headaches or neck pain, or if your brain feels "tight." Just 3 to 10 drops up to 4 times a day is all you need. This is not one for constant daily use, but just to help bring you out of a depressed state if you find yourself there.

As with any health issue, it's always good to look at your diet and lifestyle and see if there's something going on that could be improved upon. For instance, some people who suffer from depression may find that something as easy as taking more vitamin C brings relief as their body chemistry comes back into balance once again. Diet, exercise, enough sunlight, enough water — the simple stuff. But when the simple stuff just doesn't seem to cut it, it may be time to call in some herbal reinforcements. Remember, that's not always the answer. And when it isn't, it's time to talk.

Anxiety & Panic

Feeling anxious is a horrible feeling. What is supposed to be the body's way to help you flee from danger sometimes kicks into gear and won't shut down, making you feel like you're running for your life from a hungry tiger instead of dealing with an irate coworker. If you're feeling like you're on the defensive and ready to run, there are a few herbs that can offer some mental down time without knocking you out.

Perhaps you envision lemon balm (*Melissa officinalis*) as the weak decaffeinated tea your grandma drank, but then again, Grandma did know a few things. Truth be told, lemon balm can be a real anxiety reliever, even an unexpected one. A fresh plant tincture, or even a tea made from recently dried herb can bring very noticeable and surprising relief. Since lemon balm is a breeze to grown in your own garden, you can harvest a fresh batch every year for drying for your own tea, which is ideal. Dried lemon balm is less effective after it's been around a year or two, so growing your own will ensure you've always got the best. The perfect time to harvest is late spring before it flowers, preferably on a fresh, dry morning after an evening shower. But that's pretty particular, and it still works no matter when you gather it. This is quite a safe herb, so you can drink it as needed once you know your specific dosage level. As a tincture, take 30 to 40 drops up to 5 times a day. Start on the low end and work your way up to find the right dosage for you, as some people are surprised by the effect of a low dosage. Others require more for relief. It doesn't seem to coincide with weight, height, age, etc.

Hawthorn (*Crataegus spp.*) is good for the heart in more ways than one. When serious anxiety sets in, like sudden fear or even terror, hawthorn can calm you down in a hurry, and without zoning you out. Just calm. Nice. Relaxed. Like we all should be but rarely are. Whether you're a woman who's past the menopausal age and feeling anxiety and anger, something that wasn't a part of you before, or you have a sense of impending doom and start obsessing over the downturn of the economy, nuclear war, and anthrax, hawthorn is a safe and dependable friend that can be used daily, which could be a very good thing indeed, since that kind

69

of anxiety over a prolonged period of time definitely puts strain on the heart. Hawthorn is a specialist in the heart. A tincture of berries and/or flowering branches is best taken 10 to 30 drops at a time, up to 3 times a day; tea makes a nice cold infusion, 1 to 2 ounces up to 2 times a day. (**NOTE:** If you've been prescribed nitroglycerine to be taken regularly, don't take hawthorn unless you've checked with your physician and they give the okay.)

When the anxiety reaches a fevered pitch, even to the point of hysteria, valerian (*Valeriana officinalis*) can be the perfect mental slap. It brings calm and quiet to a loud and dizzy brain when you simply can't be talked out of your meltdown. This isn't one for longterm use, however, and is best used when it's really needed instead of daily. People who take valerian root over extended periods can actually find themselves feeling down and depressed. (This doesn't always happen when fresh whole plant tincture is taken instead of that from the dried root.) For bouts of hysteria, serious anxiety, and extreme worry that keeps you up at night, valerian is an amazing herbal medicine. As a tincture, either fresh whole plant or that made of the dried root, take 30 to 90 drops up to 3 times a day, or as a tea up to 2 times a day.

A more mild sedative that works well both quickly and when taken over time is celery seed (*Apium graveolens*). It doesn't offer quite the drastic results of valerian but is instead a quietness that brings peace and calm, a comfortable floating instead of a "knocked out until it passes" result. For people who have used other herbs and have found them to wear out and lose effectiveness over time, celery seed can pick up and take them through without losing its ability to calm, no matter how long someone requires its aid. Some people even claim that when taking it in the morning, it's uplifting; at night, relaxing to sleep. One half to 1 teaspoon of celery seed in hot water makes for a good medicinal tea, taken as needed. For tincture, even a mere 3 to 5 drops, 2 to 4 times a day, can work wonders.

Insomnia

I've been a bit of an insomniac my whole life. I'm not sure why that is, and it's not a constant thing, although the bouts of sleeplessness seem to be closer together the older I get. I've tried numerous remedies, some with great success and some — well, not so much. My favorite herb for insomnia is catmint (*Nepeta cataria*). I like to chew a few fresh leaves every now and then, and it's pretty good at taking the edge off a bout of stress. After a busy, overworked day when I can't seem to unplug, I find it quite useful. A little potent for chewing, bitter and an overall strange mint taste I can't quite describe, but it kind of grows on you. Especially when that flavor means I'll be "destressed" momentarily.

As a tincture, the minty weirdness is even more evident, but 20 to 40 drops in a bit of water is actually quite good; minty, a little sweet, like a mild iced tea. The first night I ever tried it, I slept like I hadn't in a long time. I woke in the morning certain it was the first time I'd opened my eyes all night. Wow, that felt great! I've been using catmint quite a bit over the last two or three years, and I still have very good results.

One nice thing about catmint is that you don't wake up feeling groggy. It's not drug-like, and you won't wake up in the middle of the night to find yourself driving your neighbor's stolen Passat to Cleveland like may happen with certain unmentionable pharmaceuticals.

And yes, catmint is actually catnip. Just don't tell kitty you're dipping into her stash for a little sleepy time help. I really don't think she'd understand.

There's no way to build up the usefulness of chamomile too much. What may sound to you like another one of your grandmother's teas is one fantastic little herb. Relaxing without hangover effects in the morning, gentle enough to drink during the day without knocking you out; for generations people have relied on its calming effects for a good night's sleep.

Here's where we pull out the big guns again — valerian (*Valeriana officinalis*). As a tea it positively stinks, and I do mean the smell. (In particular the stemmy stuff purchased commercially. If you manage to wildcraft it yourself, it's not so rank, but it looks a lot like hemlock, which is horribly poisonous! Know what you're harvesting. Always.) But boy, does valerian work! If you prefer, you can take it as a tincture or encapsulated. But remember that although valerian is a powerful natural sleep aid, even an excellent pain reliever and muscle relaxer, some people do experience a valerian "hangover" if used over time, sometimes resulting in mild depression. And unfortunately, a very few people experience exact opposite effects – valerian actually hops them up making sleep more difficult. But this isn't the norm, and I've never personally met someone who has experienced this. Consider using 30 to 90 drops of valerian tincture only when insomnia is at its worst, or when you know you'll only be relying on it for a short time.

Placing some dried lavender in your pillowcase, or even using essential oil of lavender, is often the perfect solution for those with sleep issues. Lavender oil is used in aromatherapy to calm and to aid in sleep, and it's also great for depression and anxiety relief. Some people even enjoy using dried lavender to prepare a tea before bedtime. But if you'd rather avoid taking anything internally, then simply smelling the oil or dried herb is often enough to aid in a restful night, even sweet dreams. Don't take the oil internally, however. And if applying topically, make sure it's blended with a carrier oil. Lavender oil on its own is too harsh for the skin.

If you use lavender for sleep issues, be sure to give yourself an occasional break so it doesn't wear out on you. Also, don't overdo any essential oils with young children, especially babies. Their sense of smell is much more acute than it is for adults, and what may seem mild to us may seem quite powerful to their new noses.

Although caution must often be taken no matter how natural our sleep aid, the good news is there are plenty of safe alternatives that won't leave you heavy lidded come morning. Just a few nights without sufficient sleep can be enough to throw off your health, both mentally and physically, so trying some herbs could be just what you need to cure your insomnia. The best part? You won't wake up in Cleveland.

Headaches, Earaches, & Toothaches

Pains from the neck up. Are they so distracting because they're smack in the middle of our thoughts? I'm not sure, but I do know they can get in the way of daily life. Whether it's a one-time headache because your mother-in-law has overstayed her welcome, or you suffer earaches every winter, read on, take notes, and gather herbs.

Headaches

You've had a really long day. Your toddler is letting the dog lick his granola bar, and your 12-year-old has finally decided to practice her clarinet with a broken reed - for how long? All day long you dragged around heavy laundry baskets, scrubbed green smoothie off the living room walls, and swung your little one around like a helicopter to distract him from braiding the cat. Your back hurts and so does your head. HELP!!!

73

You'll need dried yarrow (*Achillea millefolium*), boneset (*Eupatorium perfoliatum*), and skullcap (*Scutellaria lateriflora*) for the following tea mixture. (Aren't those last two appropriately named?) I suggest ordering some good organic stuff online or getting some from your local health food store, then keeping it around so it's there when you need it. Mix 1 tsp. of each herb together and place it in 2 cups of water to simmer for 30 minutes. No heavy boiling. Keep it covered too, so it doesn't evaporate too much. Strain out the herb and add just 1 tsp. of this mixture to 1 cup of hot water. You can sweeten it with honey if you prefer. Save the rest of the concoction in the fridge, or frozen as ice cubes, for later use.

This tea is a great muscle relaxer that also cleanses the blood. It'll calm those frazzled mommy nerves in no time and give you natural relief for headaches and backaches because heaven knows this whole scenario will probably be repeated again tomorrow!

Migraines

Perhaps the most common and helpful herb for the migraine is feverfew (*Tanacetum parthenium*). This is an herb that's easy to grow in your own garden, and if you harvest and dry the flowering tops and leaves, you've got all you need for the perfect medicinal tea. Unfortunately, the tea takes some getting used to for many — it's rather bitter and doesn't smell so hot either. But give it a go at the first sign of a migraine, and you'll gladly find a way to like it, no matter how it tastes. I've even chewed a couple of the plant's fresh leaves as soon as I noticed a migraine's first symptoms, and I avoided the whole nauseating experience altogether. And I have to admit I rather enjoy its bitter pungency now.

Since the tea does take time to brew and migraines are best treated right away, you might consider tincturing the plant when in season, or purchasing a bottle of the tincture to have on hand. Just 30 to 40 drops in a little water should get the job done in short order. Occasionally, a second dose might be required to end a particularly nasty round. You can take it 2 to 4 times a day. It's also a good remedy for those suffering from arthritis, fever, menstrual cramps, toothache, and stomachache.

Earaches

One of the most common health issues young children face is the earache. There are several reasons earaches are so common within the last couple of generations, including the overuse of antibiotics and bottle feeding while the baby is in a reclining position, just to name two. The earache is a discomfort any parent will want to end quickly.

My favorite remedy for earaches is St. John's-wort oil. Some health food stores do carry this, but you can make your own. St. John's-wort (*Hypericum perforatum*) is in bloom around St. John's Day, which is June 24. It's a common enough plant that grows throughout most of the U.S. and Canada, and it's easy to grow on your own, too, if you'd like to add its sunny beauty to your garden. Once you're comfortable recognizing it in the wild and you know you have a safe source, you can gather a small jar full of the yellow flowers, then cover them with olive oil or sweet almond oil. Push the flowers down into the jar with a chopstick or spoon to release as many bubbles as you can. Cap it tightly, and allow the oil to sit for a couple of weeks; some prefer to place it in a sunny window. The oil should take on a beautiful red-orange color. Strain out the plant material and store the oil in a cool, dark location. St. John's-wort oil can have a pretty decent shelf life of 2 to 3 years, but that all depends on how well you store it.

To use the oil, you can place a small amount into the sore ear by squeezing some from a cotton swab or by using a dropper, wiping away any drips from the outer ear. Pay careful attention when applying with the cotton swab, however. If the ear is already sore, the slightest bump becomes unpleasant. You also don't want to go into the ear with the swab, which could cause irreparable damage, so allow the oil to drip itself into the ear canal. The pain will often be completely knocked out in a matter of seconds to a minute, in my personal experience. I've had this stuff work with some serious wind-related ear pain, the kind that is a completely distracting ache. It's well worth the effort of growing and gathering the flowers each year. And it smells just beautiful too.

You can also try the same thing with mullein flowers (*Verbascum thapsus*). There are companies that sell mullein flower oil, both online and in brick and mortar stores, so keep your eyes peeled. Make your own in the same manner as you would for St. John's-wort.

Here's a remedy that's good for both children and adults, and since it focuses on garlic as the healing plant, you're incorporating a good dose of anti-inflammatory, anti-viral, and anti-bacterial action from the garlic. Of course, any earache accompanied by a high fever, serious pain, or any other symptoms that make that parenting radar go on alert, always consult with your doctor.

To make your own garlic oil, take about 6 cloves of garlic and chop it finely or run it through a food processor. Give it a few good whacks with the side of your cooking knife to release the oils. Make sure to use fresh garlic and not pre-chopped from the grocer's which may contain preservatives and additives. Place the garlic in a clean, dry glass jar and cover it with about a cup of fresh olive oil or sweet almond oil. Cap it tightly and allow the oil to sit for a week or two. You might opt to leave it in a sunny window for awhile. If you're in a hurry to use it, you can heat it on very low heat in a double boiler for perhaps 30 minutes; just make sure it is completely cool before use.

Once your oil has cooled, strain it thoroughly. Use a dropper to place a few drops of the oil into the ear. Hold it in place with a bit of cotton. It stays in better if you lay on your side for awhile. To remove the oil, tip the head gently to the side, catching the oil with an old clean towel. Wipe the surrounding area of the ear, but don't try to flush it out. Repeat as needed.

If you suffer from tinnitus or hearing difficulties, it is said that this may help if used over time, although it would also depend on the nature behind the tinnitus or hearing issues.

And Speaking of Tinnitus...

My grandmother always told me that if my ears were ringing, someone was thinking nice thoughts about me. If that's true, I must be more popular than Lady Gaga. My ears have been ringing constantly ever since I experienced a high fever as a small child. I'm not sure what complete silence is really like, so I'm always looking for remedies for tinnitus.

The most common reason people suffer from tinnitus is due to the prescription medication they're taking. Experiencing ringing in the ears is a common side effect, so if you have tinnitus, take a look at what's in your medicine cabinet first. If you're ready to start searching for natural remedies, here's an interesting one that may just work for you: onion juice. For many who have tried it, a few drops of onion juice placed in each ear can get rid of tinnitus while improving hearing.

If you have tinnitus, you should also examine your diet. Oftentimes too much caffeine or salt, or eating processed foods can kick up or cause tinnitus, so stay as chemical free as possible and eat plenty of those fresh fruits and vegetables. See? Your mom was right. Eat your vegetables.

Meniere's Disease

There's still a lot to learn about treating Meniere's disease naturally. That's partially because it's a tough one to diagnose. Talk to three different doctors, and they'll give you three different lists of symptoms. (Talk to three different Meniere's patients, however, and they'll probably all say pretty much the same thing.) It's pretty exciting that there are so many natural options to try, so if you've been diagnosed with it, see what works best for you and your symptoms.

Ground ivy (*Nepeta hederacea*) is one of those plants that shows up everywhere, and most people would deem it a weed. But I don't. It's got so many great and varied uses that I see it as an amazing helper. Funny, but it seems the most common of weeds are usually the most helpful. Perhaps that's why we trip over them at every turn. They're just begging to be used. Ground ivy is great for ear issues including tinnitus and inner ear problems such as Meniere's. A tincture works quite well if applied topically to the base of the skull and along the sides of the neck where you feel the most deeply set discomfort. Since the inner ear is so difficult to get to, applying a few drops at the surface of wherever you feel deep down pain and tightness can really help ease a very uncomfortable experience. Ground ivy is pretty safe, so you can apply several drops to the area without worries. Taking it internally can help too — 20 to 40 drops up to 4 times daily — but in all honesty, it works much faster used as a topical. When you're truly uncomfortable, that can make all the difference.

Another helpful topical for people with Meniere's is juniper oil. A good essential oil of juniper (*Juniperus communis*) can be applied to the temples during bouts of vertigo. Or if you happen to have a lot of the aforementioned ground ivy in dried form, you can make a ground ivy tea, also a remedy for vertigo.

Many people with Meniere's describe a strange sensation in the brain, saying it feels "tight." This can be a totally distracting symptom, and although not usually painful, people who experience it would certainly like to get rid of it, and fast. Mullein root may be just the thing. Mullein (*Verbascum thapsis*), a common plant found in wasteland areas, roadsides, abandoned farmer's fields, etc., has a whole host of uses. Each part of the plant (as with many herbs) offers something different and unique from the other parts. In this case, the root of the mullein plant is an excellent relaxer. Great for tight muscles and back pain, it also has the ability to release the tight sensation that sufferers of Meniere's often experience. Many express the wonderful release of the symptom and a feeling of the mind opening. I've felt this myself every time I've had mullein root tea, and it's pretty impressive.

Unfortunately, mullein root is virtually impossible to come by in commerce, but it's so readily available in such a wide variety of regions that you can dig it up yourself if you're comfortable in identifying the plant. Since you are using the root here, it's most important to make sure that the area is clean. No digging it up off the side of the highway, for instance, which more than likely contains contaminated soil. Stick to nice, big open fields where you can freely dig without getting arrested for weed swiping, etc. No one likes to have their tall, furry weeds stolen.

The root can be tinctured, dried for tea, or made into a tea when still fresh, and you can dig up the roots anytime of year, even during the winter. I always like to dig them up in spring and fall, but I've also gathered some during other times of the year and found the roots worked well, anyway. For the tincture, try 30 to 50 drops up to 4 times a day. With the tea, whether from dried or fresh root, prepare a strong decoction and take 2 or 3 ounces up to 4 times a day.

One big problem with Meniere's is the inflammation of the inner ear which causes the pain and ringing, and eventually the hearing loss. Having a good anti-inflammatory on your side is indispensable. Turmeric (*Curcuma longa*) is one of the best I know, and you can get this one just about anywhere, even fresh in grocery stores. Some people prefer turmeric capsules, but I'll take a good fresh root tincture any day. Too often, any herb placed into capsules and sold are all stems and twigs, and old, dusty herbs that have been sitting around way too long. But get some turmeric tincture from a health food store, or better yet, make your own from fresh root, and you've got one terrific anti-inflammatory to use. Thirty to 40 drops taken in some water can knock out that inner ear inflammation pain in about 10 to 15 minutes. Taken every day, you can help stave off the inflammation before it occurs, and without all the nasty side effects of over-the-counter anti-inflammatories. (Liver transplants are no fun, or so I am told.) Feel free to use this remedy for any inflammation you need to get a handle on.

Toothaches

Few body pains are as horrible as the toothache. We've all had them – you can't sleep, you can't eat; you pretty much just sit or pace, let it throb, and hope the dentist wants to come in on a Sunday afternoon to take an emergency peek. (How come the pain only occurs on weekends and holidays, anyway?) If you find yourself experiencing the terrible toothache, here are few natural remedies that you might try.

We're supposing if you have a nasty toothache you probably won't be going far from home anyway, so you might as well give garlic a shot. Peel a garlic clove, give it a nice little squish with your teeth, and place it right on the sore tooth or in the cavity.

This next one is actually good for teething babies as well. If you have a baby, consider keeping a bottle of clove oil around the house at all times. First off, make sure what you have is the real deal and not clove flavoring sometimes used in cooking. Moisten a bit of cotton with the oil, then place directly on the affected tooth, being careful not to get too much on the gums as it can be slightly irritating to some. Try not to use much with children since it's strong, and they might revolt from you trying it again if you go too heavy handed the first time. I recommend trying it on yourself first to get an idea of how much you think they'd be able to handle.

Many people swear by the following remedy. Simply add sea salt to warm water to make a heavily salted solution. Rinse your mouth repeatedly by holding the water in your mouth and sloshing it around for as long as you can. This also helps irritated gums and abscessed teeth.

Here's one that works just as with the garlic. Cut and peel a small chunk of fresh ginger and chew it if you can. Some people find this to be too strong and spicy of a remedy, but if you can handle it, you'll be glad you gave it a shot. (Chewing raw ginger is also great for upset stomachs, morning sickness, and coughing spells.)

An herbalist hero of mine, Michael Moore of the Southwest School of Botanical Medicine, told the following story as part of his distance learning program. When stopping in a bar in Arkansas, he spotted a large jar next to the alcohol bottles. The jar was filled with what looked like roots, and he asked the bartender what it was. The bartender told him they were yarrow roots (*Achillea millefolium*), and that they'd been preserved in brandy. Anyone with a toothache was welcome to have a yarrow root for chewing on. The locals swore by this remedy and would stop by for a root whenever serious tooth pain struck. Michael said he'd never heard of this remedy anywhere else in his years of herbalism, but it fascinated him. I've not tried it yet myself, but I'm currently growing some yarrow so I can dig it up and steep some in brandy, just in case. I want to see if those Arkansas bartenders really know what they're talking about.

Keep these toothache remedies in mind and on hand, and tell that dentist you'll see him Monday instead.

Preparing Herbal Teas for Medicinal Use

As we've been discovering on our trek through this book, herbs are fantastic and varied alternative medicines when used properly, and they're so much more fun than anything over the counter. For the most part, they're inexpensive compared to the average pharmaceutical, and with some online shopping, or even hunting your local flora, there's almost nothing that isn't available to the home herbalist. But what you may not realize is that simply plunking a dried-up tea bag in a mug of hot water isn't quite the best way to take advantage of an herb's medicinal values.

To prepare a dried herb, it's best to make sure it's finely chopped or ground to a coarse powder. Use a spare coffee grinder just for herbs and spices. (If you clean it well after every use, you won't have to worry about flavors from your last batch of celery seed getting into everything else that follows.) Fresh herbs can be cut into small pieces with some kitchen scissors; leaves and flowers can be bruised or crushed a little, perhaps with a mortar and pestle, or a spoon in a bowl; fresh roots should be cut into thin slices or little chunks.

The water you use should be purified, soft, or distilled if possible. Some people even collect rainwater, which sounds fantastic if you live in a clean environment. (Smoggy-city dwellers may think twice on this one.) For larger batches that will be consumed over the course of a day or two, water should be heated to almost boiling and 1 pint (500 ml) should be placed in a glass, earthenware, or porcelain container. There are infusion pots that work best for preparing herb teas by suspending the herb towards the top of the hot water, but you can also wing it if you don't have an infusion pot. I use a tea ball, half filled with herb, that I hang towards the top of the water by holding the tea ball chain in place with the lid of the pot. (Always make sure you cover the tea with a lid.) By keeping the herb towards the top of the teapot, you are causing the water molecules to drag the herb's properties to the bottom of the pot. More "empty" water molecules rise to the top, taking the herbal properties back to the bottom. It's all a matter of gravity, and it will pull the most out of your herb.

For a simple mug of tea, approximately 1 teaspoon of herb is generally used. (I've specified throughout this book when appropriate.) Again, try and suspend the tea ball or tea bag towards the top of the mug, and cover. With tea bags, it's helpful to wrap the string around the mug handle to hold the tea bag towards the top. Then cover the mug with a small plate or whatever you can snag that will fit.

Here's the part most people don't realize: Hot tea used for medicinal purposes are best left to steep for 20 to 30 minutes, not the usual 3 to 5 minutes as one would for a beverage tea. After your wait is up, remove the herb, squish out all the water, and add more water to the pot to make sure it still equals about 1 pint (500 ml.) when making the larger batches. It's okay and even beneficial if there are bits of herb floating in your tea – and it looks cool and earthy too -- so don't strain it unless you're really bothered by drinking tea with floaties.

Cold infusions are teas prepared by pre-moistening the herb with water, wrapping it in cheesecloth or placing it in a tea ball, then adding 32 parts room temperature water by volume (1 ounce of herb plus 32 ounces of water, etc.) The tea sits overnight and is then strained. Add enough water to bring the tea back to its original amount.

Strong decoctions are often used with roots, barks, or woody herbs. In this case, the herb is placed in a pan in 32 parts water on the stovetop. Heat the water slowly to the boiling point, then boil for 10 minutes before allowing to cool slightly and straining out the herb. Again, add enough water to bring the tea back up to its original volume.

The average adult dosage for most herbal teas is one cup three times daily, but the different teas do vary, so check the more specific notations in this book to be certain. I've also added as much dosage info as possible on the Herbal Medicine Chest section at the end of this book. You can keep your unused tea for about 24 hours if stored in the fridge, but don't go beyond that or you'll start losing the benefits.

In the end, don't sweat it if you don't have the right infusion pot or a 1-pint jar or a tea ball. Your great grandmother probably just tossed a teaspoon of herb in a mug, put a small plate on top, and let it steep. After her 20 to 30 minute wait (she probably guesstimated), she'd strain the stuff back out with a spoon and serve it up – beautiful earthy floaties and all!

Making a Simple Tincture

Not every herb can be tinctured, but most of them we've talked about can be. The beauty of the tincture is that it's easy to take, it's easy to make, and it stores for a very long time — 10 years or longer for most. Many people find it rather intimidating at first, but it really isn't; and there is an easy way to go about it. Once you've made one tincture, you'll want to make more. I have storage shelves loaded with the stuff to prove it. All those bottles lined up on a shelf can make you feel pretty darned self sufficient, knowing you're able to provide some homemade family medicinals.

For tinctures, you need a clean jar with a tight-fitting lid, fresh herbs (occasionally dried), and alcohol.

Let's start with the jar, shall we? I save pasta sauce jars. They tend to have lids with a sort of built-in gasket already. Pickle jars are great too. Just be sure they're washed out thoroughly, and that you store them with the lid off. Otherwise, when you're ready to use your "clean" jar, you might open it to a burst of pickle or garlic aroma. Give a quick rinse before using, and you're all set.

For the herbs, sometimes we use the flowering tops (the top 2 to 3 inches of the plant), the entire plant, or the roots. Other times we use all three parts in what would be called a "whole plant tincture." I've let you know throughout the book, and in the Herbal Medicine Chest list at the end, what part to use of which plant when tincturing was mentioned.

For the alcohol, you have a few options here. In some states, the good grain alcohol that's 190 proof isn't legal, which is unfortunate for the herbalist since the higher proofs pull out more plant constituents than lower proofs. So unless your Uncle Buck has a still hidden out in the woods somewhere, you'll probably have to settle for some good old vodka. Get the highest proof you can, the cheapest brand you can, and lock it up as tight as you can if you've got kids, or perhaps a spouse who likes vodka and Coke after work and might not mind skimming off your stash when you're not looking.

We're going to use the Simpler's method because it's — well, simple. Personally, I often make tinctures by using my fancy kitchen scale, referring to notes from years gone by, checking up on what other herbalists deem successful, etc. But in the end, your great grandmother probably didn't do any of that either, and you don't really need to most of the time. Will it be the very finest quality with consistent results year after year? Not necessarily. But, then, even the best measurers and research-loving herbalists experience differences from one year to the next. After all, the plant will grow how the plant will grow. It will be a little different each year, anyway, depending on rainfall, soil quality, etc. Plants don't like to do all that measuring stuff when they grow.

For the Simpler's method, you chop up your fresh herb or root well, pack it down in the jar, but not tightly, and fill the jar with the alcohol of your choosing until the plant material is fully covered with a little to spare. If it floats, you can put a flat stone on top, but then make sure you never shake the jar or it'll break. Cap the jar off tightly.

At this point, you could use a bit of folded plastic wrap over the mouth of the jar before adding the lid. Yes, I realize plastic wrap isn't very environmentally friendly. Perhaps you could reuse it to death and then recycle it; then feel guilt-ridden for a significant period of time. You may have a better solution, though, or if you're really fortunate, you already have a nice shelf of unused canning jars in the basement that you didn't ever know what to do with — until now.

Once the jar is filled and capped, give it a gentle shake, unless you put a stone on top of the herbs. Then slap a label on it that says the name of the herb, the date, what kind of alcohol you used, and perhaps where you picked the herb so you remember for future years. And maybe a picture of you holding herbs, or "Made by Beth," etc. Go ahead — personalize it! You made medicine all by yourself and you should be proud.

You don't need to shake the jar or tip it anymore. The alcohol will extract everything out of the herbs if left to its own devices. After awhile, you'll notice the plant material will lose its color as the alcohol gains color. Store in a dark location for 2 to 4 weeks (even more if you feel like it. It won't hurt), then carefully strain the plant material out of the tincture. I use a ricer, which serves to both strain the herb and press out the alcohol, thus losing much less than if you simply strained it, or, say, squeezed it out with your bare hands. So far, it's the best way I've found for getting that last little bit out without wearing me down, twisting cheese cloth around, etc., as many tend to do.

Now you can pour the tincture back into the jar and cap it tightly once again. At this point, you can choose to store smaller amounts in 1-ounce amber dropper bottles for travel or ease of use.

How to Make Salve

Salve is one of those really rewarding things because when you make it, you don't usually walk away with just one tin. You instead end up with several, and since that's way more than most of us can use in a couple of years' time, that means you have the great opportunity to share your stuff. Since salve is more familiar to people than tinctures, for instance, they're more than happy to enjoy your herbal offerings and will immediately uncap it, smell it, and rub it on. It's a pretty satisfying thing to share something healthy that you've made with friends and family.

Salve isn't difficult, although I think it often intimidates people, as does tincture making. Although there are several steps to it, it only takes one try to understand the whole process, and more than likely, to get hooked on doing it.

I'd recommend getting yourself the proper tools first and setting them aside for salve making only. There are countless ways to go about this, so I'll just tell you how I do it and what I use, since I don't use any fancy equipment. You probably already have everything you need:

An old saucepan, about a 3-quart
Glass measuring cup, preferably anything larger than 1 cup
Beeswax (grated, pastilles, etc. If you have to grate it yourself, plan for plenty of extra time.)
Sweet almond oil (I prefer food grade) *or* olive oil (this does alter the fragrance, however)
Vitamin E capsules, natural (These are not only good for the skin, but aid as natural preservative.)
Small heat-proof glass jars, tins, etc., with lids
Herbs and/or essential oils of your choosing

Chop your fresh herbs or grind your dried herbs, and place them in a jar large enough to fit all the herbs when packed loosely into the jar. Cover the herbs with the oil completely and push out all the air bubbles with a wooden chopstick or other handy utensil. Place a cap on the jar and give the jar a couple of gentle thunks on the countertop. Not enough to break your jar, mind you; just enough to knock out a few more air bubbles. Keeping the air out will keep that oil fresher while it sits.

Now the hard part: Wait about 2 weeks. Some people place their oil jar in a sunny window, others don't. I like the sunny window approach because it allows it to steep, and there's something kind of magical about telling yourself your salve will contain some sunshine. Just don't allow the jar to get too hot. The oil and the plant material (especially when using fresh herbs) can start to spoil if it sits too long, or if it gets too hot.

After you've made it through a couple of weeks of staring at your jar and anticipating salve-like goodness, you can finally make your salve. Dump the oil, herbs and all, into your large glass measuring cup.

Fold a paper towel in fourths and place it in the bottom of your pan, then place the measuring cup in the pan. (Just a little precaution here so the cup won't bounce around and break if the water accidentally starts to boil.) Add water to the pan (NOT the measuring cup holding the oil) so that when you place the measuring cup in the pan, it rests on the paper towel and is surrounded with water. Now place the pan on very, very low heat. When the water gets hot and is NOT boiling or simmering, let the oil and herbs steep for about 30 minutes, keeping a close eye on both the water level and the oil. You don't want the oil to boil or simmer at all. And don't boil it. Or simmer. Or boil.

Now turn off the heat, allow the oil to cool, and strain out the herbs. An old mesh colander is a good choice. Pour the strained oil back into the glass measuring cup, and place the cup back into the pan, making sure there's still plenty of water in there. It works best if the water on the outside is at least level with the oil on the inside. This will help melt your beeswax better.

Heat the oil back up and add your beeswax. The easiest way to figure out how much beeswax to add is to use about 1/6 the amount of oil. So, for instance, if you have 6 ounces of oil, you'd need to start with 1 ounce of beeswax. It's always best to guess on the low side because we can adjust this easily later on.

Once all the beeswax has dissolved, take a spoon and put a few drops of the salve onto a small plate. Wait for it to cool so you can see if it's the consistency you'd like. (Stick the plate in your freezer for about 30 seconds if you're impatient.) If it's too goopy or thin, add more beeswax, repeating the testing process until it's where you like it. If you know you'll be adding essential oil to the salve, be sure to make allowances for that by keeping the salve only slightly firmer than desired.

Turn off the heat, squeeze in the contents of a few Vitamin E caps, (I use one capsule per every 4 oz. of salve), and add the essential oil, if required. While the oil mixture is still warm, pour directly into your containers. Allow them all to cool while uncapped. When the bottoms of the containers are completely cool to the touch, you can cap everything and label them. Make sure to add the name of the salve, the herbs you used, and a date.

Be sure that the salve is stored in a cool, dark place. The better you are about that, the longer it will last.

93

Herbal Medicine Chest

This section lists all the herbs discussed throughout Herbs Gone Wild. It also gives dosage ranges for tinctures and teas. This is not an all-encompassing list meant to cover every usage of the plant, but rather, to give you an overview of what was discussed in this book. Teas below are standard infusions (herbs allowed to steep in hot water before straining) unless otherwise specified.

For dosages, start out at the low end and work your way up to where the herbs give you the best results. **For children, see the conversion at the bottom of this list.** Always tell your doctor what you're taking.

Aloe (*Aloe vera*) Gel from leaves. Topical as needed.

Anemone (*Anemone hirsutissima*) Whole fresh plant. Tincture: 3 – 10 drops to 4x daily.

Balsamroot (*Balsamorhiza*) Root. Tincture: 20 – 50 drops to 4x daily.

Black Walnut (*Juglans major*) Leaves. Tincture: 30 – 90 drops to 3x daily. Tea: 2 – 4 oz. to 3x daily.

Boneset (*Eupatorium perfoliatum*) Flowering herb. Tincture: 20 – 40 drops in hot water, to 4x daily. Tea: 2 – 6 oz. to 3x daily.

Burdock (*Arctium lappa*) Root. 30 – 90 drops to 3x daily. Tea: 2 – 4 oz. to 3x daily.

Cardamom (*Elettaria cardamomum*) Seeds. Suck or chew 1 – 2 seeds as needed. Tincture: 30 – 40 drops to 5x daily.

Catmint (*Nepeta cataria*) Flowering herb. 20 – 40 drops to 3x daily.

Cayenne (*Capsicum*) Fruit. Tincture: 5 – 15 drops in water or capsule to 5x daily, or topically as needed.

Celery (*Apium graveolens*) Seeds. Tincture: 3 – 30 drops to 4x daily. Tea: ½ – 1 tsp. seed steeped in hot water, as needed.

Chamomile (*Matricaria recutita*) Flowers. Tincture: 30 – 40 drops to 5x daily. Tea: 2 – 4 oz. as needed.

Cinnamon (*Cinnamomum verum*) Bark. Tincture: 20 – 50 drops to 4x daily. Tea: 2 – 4 oz. to 4x daily.

Cinquefoil (*Potentilla*) Whole plant. Tea as part of compress mixture.

Cleavers (*Galium aparine*) Whole plant. Tincture: 1 – 2 tsp. to 4x daily. Juice of fresh plant: ½ – 1 tsp. to 4x daily.

Clove (*Caryophyllus*) Essential oil of unripe buds placed on a cotton ball and put either directly on or in affected tooth; avoid gums if possible.

Comfrey (*Symphytum officinale*) Leaf or root. Tea (cold infusion): 2 – 6 oz. of leaf tea or 1 – 4 oz. of root tea, to 3x daily. Short-term use only.

Dandelion (*Taraxacum officinale*) Root and/or leaf. Tincture (root) : ½ – 1 tsp. to 4x daily. Tea (root, strong decoction): 2 – 4 oz. to 4x daily. Tea (leaf): 3 – 4 oz. as needed.

Echinacea (*Echinacea angustifulium* or *purpurea*) Root and flowers. Tincture: 30 – 100 drops as needed. Tea (cold infusion): 2 – 4 oz to 5x daily.

Elder (*Sambucus nigra* or *canadensis*) Flowers or leaves. Tea (flowers): 2 – 4 oz. to 3x daily. Tea (leaves, cold infusion): 1 – 2 oz. to 3x daily.

Elecampane (*Inula helenium*) Root. Tincture: 10 – 30 drops to 4x daily. Tea (strong decoction): 2 – 6 oz. to 3x daily.

Eyebright (*Euphrasia officinalis*) Whole herb. Tincture: 30 – 90 to 4x daily. Tea (strong decoction): 2 – 4 oz. to 4x daily. Can also be used on a compress or topically as an eyewash.

Fennel (*Foeniculum vulgare*) Seed. Tincture: 30 – 60 drops in warm water, as needed. Tea: as needed.

Feverfew (*Tanacetum parthenium*) Flowering herb. Tea: 1 – 4 oz. as needed; for short-term use only.

Flax (*Linum*) Seed. Fresh ground only, 1 – 2 tsp. sprinkled on food or stirred into beverage.

Garlic (*Allium sativum*) Bulb. Eat fresh or grind for poultice. Tincture: 15 – 40 drops to 3x daily.

Goldenrod (*Solidago spp.*) Whole herb. Tincture: 30 – 40 drops to 5x daily. Tea: 1 – 3 oz. to 5x daily.

Goldenseal (*Hydrastis*) Root and leaf. Tincture: 20 – 40 drops to 4x daily. Not suited to tea.

Goldthread (*Coptis*) Root and herb. Tincture: 30 – 60 drops to 3x daily; topically as needed. Tea (strong decoction): topically as needed.

Ground Ivy (*Nepeta hederacea*) Whole plant. Tincture: 20 – 40 drops to 4x daily. Tea: 4 – 6 oz. to 4x daily.

Hawthorn (*Crataegus spp.*) Flowering branches and/or berries. Tincture: 10 – 30 drops to 3x daily. Tea (cold infusion): 1 – 2 oz. to 2x daily.

Hibiscus (*Hibiscus sabdariffa*) Dried flowers. Tea: 6 – 8 oz. up to 2x daily.

Horehound (*Marrubium*) Flowering herb. Tincture: 30 – 90 drops to 4x daily. Tea (cold infusion): 2 – 4 oz. to 4x daily.

Horse Nettle (*Solanum carolinense*) Root. Tincture: 10 – 40 drops occasionally; not for regular use.

Horseradish (*Armoracia*) Fresh grated root. ½ – 1 ½ tsp. internally (with honey if preferred) or used externally in cup of hand, held over mouth and nose.

Immortal (*Asclepias asperula*) Root. Tincture: 5 – 30 drops to 3x daily.

Jewelweed (*Impatiens capensis*) Fresh plant, juiced, for topical. Or prepare salve from fresh plant. Use as needed.

Juniper (*Juniperus communis*) Berries. Tincture: 20 – 40 drops to 3x daily. Tea: 2 – 3 oz. to 3x daily. Short term use only, if using internally; no more than 6 consecutive weeks usage. Essential oil: Topically, blended with carrier oil such as sweet almond or olive, as needed.

Lavender (*Lavandula spp.*) Flowers. Tea: 2 – 3 oz. to 4x daily. Essential oil: Topically, blended with carrier oil such as sweet almond or olive, as needed.

Lemon Balm (*Melissa officinalis*) Flowering herb. Tincture: 30 – 40 drops to 5x daily. Tea: as needed.

Licorice (*Glycyrrhiza glabra*) Root. Tincture: 30 – 40 drops to 5x daily. Tea: 1 – 3 oz. to 3x daily. Can cause sodium retention, so take for no longer than 4 weeks.

Milkweed, Common (*Asclepias cornuta*) Root. 5 – 30 drops to 3x daily.

Motherwort (*Leonurus cardiaca*) Flowering herb. Tincture: 30 – 60 drops to 4x daily. Tea: 2 – 4 oz. to 4x daily.

Mullein (*Verbascum thapsis*) Root, leaf, or flower. Tincture, all forms: 30 – 90 drops to 4x daily. Tea: Strong decoction for root, 2 – 3 oz. to 4x daily. Standard infusion for leaves, 2 – 3 oz. to 4x daily.

Osha (*Ligusticum porter*) Root. Tincture: 20 – 60 drops to 3x daily. For more acute infections, congestion, etc., take 60 – 120 drops every 2 hrs. until symptoms subside. Tea: 6 – 8 oz. to 3x daily.

Ox-Eye Daisy (*Chrysanthemum leucanthemum*) Tea: 6 – 8 oz. to 4x daily.

Parsley (*Petroselinum*) Fresh. Take internally as needed.

Passionflower (*Passiflora incarnate*) Whole herb. Tincture: ½ – 1 ½ tsp. to 4x daily. Tea: 2 – 6 oz. to 4x daily.

Pepper, Black (*Piper nigrum*) Peppercorns. Used as breath freshener; suck on peppercorn for as long as needed, then spit out.

Peppermint (*Mentha piperita*) Whole herb. Tea: as needed.

Pipsissewa (*Chimaphila*) Whole herb. Tincture: 20 – 50 drops to 4x daily. Tea: 4 – 8 oz. to 4x daily.

Plantain (*Plantago major*) Fresh leaves. Ground or crushed for poultice, or prepared in a salve. Topically as needed.

Ragweed (*Ambrosia*) Whole herb. Tincture: 20 – 40 drops to 4x daily. Tea: 1 – 2 oz. to 4x daily.

Raspberry (*Rubus idaeus*) Leaves. Tea: Take as needed.

Rose Hips (*Rosaceae*) Tea: Take as needed.

Rosemary (*Rosemarinus officinalis*) Leaves. Tea: 2 – 4 oz. as needed.

Sage (*Salvia*) Flowering herb. Tincture: 30 – 60 drops as needed. Tea: 2 – 4 oz. as needed.

Senna (*Cassia marilandica*) Leaves, Tea: 4 – 8 oz. taken in evening for morning relief. Or soak 10 – 15 pods in water for 30 min. before drinking. Not for daily use.

Shepherd's Purse (*Capsella bursa-pastoris*) Whole plant. Tea: Use as needed for a compress.

Skullcap (*Scutellaria lateriflora*) Whole herb. Tincture: 20 – 60 drops to 3x daily. Tea: 2 – 6 oz. to 3x daily.

Slippery Elm (*Ulmus rubra*) Powdered bark. Gruel: Taken 1 – 3x daily, as needed.

Solomon's Seal, False or True (*Polygonatum multiflorum* or *Smilacina racemosa*) Tincture: 20 – 30 drops to 3x daily; or topically as needed.

Stinging Nettle (*Urtica dioica*) Whole herb. Tea: Taken as needed.

St. Johns Wort (*Hypericum perforatum*) Flowering herb. Tincture: 20 – 30 drops to 3x daily. Tea: 3 – 6 oz. to 3x daily. However, fresh plant tincture is the superior form.

Turmeric (*Curcuma longa*) Root. Tincture: 30 – 40 drops to 5x daily.

Valerian (*Valeriana officinalis*) Whole plant. Tincture: 30 – 90 drops to 3x daily. Tea: 4 – 6 oz. as needed. Neither form is meant for regular, daily usage.

White Pine (*Pinus strobus*) Bark or whole new growth, needles removed. Tea: 6 – 8 oz. as needed.

Wild Oat (*Avena sativa*) Unripe fresh seed. Tincture: 10 – 20 drops to 4x daily. Tea: dry but green stems, 4 – 8 oz. to 4x daily.

Witch Hazel (*Hamamelis*) Twigs and leaves. Tincture or astringent: topically as needed.

Wormwood (*Artemisia absinthium*) Dried plant. External use as needed for Vinegar of the Four Thieves.

Yarrow (*Achillea millefolium*) Whole flowering plant. Tincture: 10 – 40 drops to 5x daily. Tea: 2 – 4 oz. to 5x daily.

Yerba Mansa (*Anemopsis*) Root. Tincture: 15 – 30 drops to 1 oz. distilled water and 1 oz. glycerin as a throat spray to be used as needed. Refrigerate between uses. Lasts 2 – 3 days.

Converting Dosages for Children: Clark's Rule

To figure out how much herbal medicine to give a child, you divide the child's weight in pounds by 150. This will give you an approximate fraction of the adult dose. For instance, for a 50-pound child, you'd end up with 50/150, or a ⅓ dose. As an adult may require 30 drops of tincture taken 3 times a day, a child receiving the same medicine would receive 10 drops of tincture 3 times a day.

Always use your very best judgment in administering these or any alternative therapies to children. Remember to consult with your health care professional before treating your child, and if you or your child are taking prescription medications, always check with your doctor before adding herbal remedies.

Conclusion

I sincerely hope this walk through herbalism has been a fruitful one for you, and that it's just the beginning of your journey back to a more natural lifestyle. This world is so busy, and our lives so hectic, that it's too easy to lose touch with our roots. And our roots are natural and go deep.

I always like to back up a moment and look at the big picture. In this case, that means remembering our grandmothers throughout time. That is a pretty big picture, isn't it? But try, if you can, to visualize that long line of women who belong to you, whether you know their names or not. Throughout human history, they've been treating their families in whatever way they knew how. They loved their families fiercely, just like you do. And, just like you, they'd do whatever it took to keep them healthy and safe. While modern medicine hasn't been readily available to the masses for very long at all, plants have been around for even longer than our grandmothers. They don't require a health care plan or an insurance card. They've been there all along, with healing in their leaves and blooms, their roots and stems.

Is it any wonder, then, that even during this hectic age, we often find some sense of peace and deep satisfaction by turning back the hands of time, heading for the deep forest or the open field, and gathering the same plants our grandmothers rested their hands upon for thousands of years? I think it all makes perfect sense. Our grandmothers would want us to know.

Contact Me

Do you have an herbal remedy of your own? Perhaps something your mother or grandmother used, something you discovered, or a plant you just can't live without? Or perhaps you tried a remedy in this book and you have a story you'd like to share with me about your experience. Maybe your anecdote or suggestion will even be included in a future book! I'd love to hear from you.

themommyspot@gmail.com

Author's Website: http://www.DianeKidman.com

Acknowledgements

A thousand thanks to all who helped me to complete this project. Thanks to the Southwest School of Botanical Medicine and herbalists Michael Moore and Donna Chesner for giving me a good pair of herbalist's wings; to the kind people at Madcap Coffee and the Grand Rapids Art Museum who let me hang out and type furiously while in their inspiring surroundings; to my son who teaches me more than I teach him; and most especially to my husband, whose ever present faith in me is just one more reason I love him.

CPSIA information can be obtained at www.ICGtesting.com
Printed in the USA
LVOW10s1614280414

383557LV00016B/658/P